SHORT-TERM PSYCHOTHERAPY AND EMOTIONAL CRISIS

Short-Term Psychotherapy and

Emotional Crisis   PETER E. SIFNEOS

HARVARD UNIVERSITY PRESS
CAMBRIDGE, MASSACHUSETTS, AND LONDON, ENGLAND

TO HELENE J. LUCAS SIFNEOS

Journaliste féministe
Ecrivain philanthrope
Tante bien aimée

FOREWORD

Few things are more frightening to man than man himself. As Freud first showed in a systematic way, the irrational elements of the human mind are unsurpassed in their capacity to arouse terror, and the individual must be spared a full conscious recognition of them if he is to preserve his peace of mind, not to say his sanity. It is not surprising, therefore, that the scientist who chooses to focus his attention on man's inner life of feeling and fantasy is often an object of suspicion and that the therapeutic approaches resulting from his insights are frequently disparaged.

There is hardly a criticism that has not been leveled at psychotherapy: it is ineffective; it is dangerous; it is too limited, too long, too expensive; carried on in the secrecy of the consulting room, its techniques remain arcana unavailable to scientific scrutiny; all psychotherapeutic methods are equally efficacious, and there are no valid grounds for choosing one over another; studies of outcome are uncontrolled and provide no evidence that it has value; psychotherapy is nothing but common sense, or nonsense, or fraud.

The dedicated psychotherapist is undaunted by these frequently contradictory comments. He knows from his own experience that his treatment methods work, and he is aware that the demand for rigorous proof comes from those who like their world to be an orderly place and expect natural phenomena to conform to the clear definitions and sharply delineated categories of ideal reason. God is less obsessional, and the real world of creation is full of stubborn facts that refuse to be marshalled or quantified; nowhere is this more true than in the realm of human subjective experience and the psychology that studies it.

And yet the criticisms do have a certain justification. Too often the psychotherapist is content to rely on his intuitive convictions alone. Disheartened by the complexity of the variables that confront him, impatient with the harness of scientific method, he shies away from any attempt to define his procedures or to validate his claims of success. A notable few, however, have refused to be dismayed by the difficulties inherent in a scientific study of psychotherapy. Fully recognizing that their questions must be inexact and their answers tentative, they have sought to gain more systematic information about its nature, to search for shorter and more effective procedures, and to examine the results of their application. Among them is the author of this book.

Based on his many years of experience with brief psychotherapy in an outpatient setting, Dr. Sifneos' volume deals with the criteria for selecting patients, the definition and description of his therapeutic techniques, the process of therapy as it is experienced by the patients themselves, and the effectiveness of treatment as determined by controlled experiment and careful followup studies of outcome. What particularly sets this book apart from others of its genre is the author's copious use of clinical material from recorded therapeutic sessions. His illustrative cases richly illuminate his exposition of fact and theory and simultaneously allow the reader to see a highly skilled therapist at work with his patients — a privilege that is to be valued by beginner and expert alike. A major contribution to psychiatric practice and knowledge, *Short-Term Psychotherapy and Emotional Crisis* deserves the wide audience to whom it is addressed.

John C. Nemiah, M.D.
Boston, December 1971

PREFACE

This book is about a specialized kind of psychotherapy the main features of which are: brevity, emotional reeducation, problem-solving, and limited goals. For lack of a better term it is called "anxiety provoking" because an attempt is made to increase anxiety in order to bring about these goals.

Misunderstandings have resulted from the use of various terms referring to psychotherapy such as, for example, "insight," "intensive," "psychoanalytically oriented," and "dynamic." Furthermore, it is well known that the majority of psychiatrists consider "long-term psychotherapy" as the treatment of choice for most patients suffering from psychoneurotic disorders. This old and well-entrenched attitude, which tends to view the therapist as indispensable to his patient, has been responsible, by and large, for the resistance encountered by those who have tried to shorten the length of psychotherapy and for the prevailing confusion about the use of the terms "brief," "crisis oriented," and "short-term" psychotherapy. Although the short term interval is the only element which a variety of therapeutic techniques have in common with each other, they are usually considered to be identical and are largely ignored. In most of the psychiatry facilities the severity of the patient's complaints plays, invariably, the determining role in the decision to offer him long-term psychotherapy, while on the "waiting list" are those individuals whose difficulties are considered to be "mild" or of "secondary importance."

Some investigators, stimulated by the scientific trend in psychiatry, have tried to develop special kinds of short-term psychotherapy — not for economic reasons, not as a second-best alternative to long-term psychotherapy or psychoanalysis, not as a means of challenging their colleagues, and not as a way to urge them to get out of their constricted state of inertia, but primarily because they are convinced that these shorter psychotherapeutic techniques offer the best opportunity to meet the needs of selected groups of patients with mild and at times more severe psychiatric difficulties.

In my opinion, there should be no confusion about the role of short-term psychotherapies. They are valuable additions to the psychiatrists' armamentarium because they offer the best help to patients who, unable to deal with their emotional crises, have developed a variety of fairly well circumscribed psychoneurotic illnesses.

Is, then, the introduction of yet another term such as "anxiety-provoking" necessary? Will it add to the general confusion? It is hoped that this will not be the case, because the term is used simply for communication purposes. It is also used to define and describe specifically the technique which we used and which is based on the following model: Out of a variety of presenting complaints the patient is asked to assign top priority to the one emotional problem which he wants to overcome. The therapist, who acts as both evaluator and teacher can obtain, by skillful interviewing and history-taking, enough information from the patient to enable him to set up a tentative psychodynamic hypothesis to help him arrive at a formulation of the emotional conflicts underlying the patient's difficulty. Throughout the treatment he concentrates his attention especially on these conflicts in an effort to help the patient to learn a new way to solve his emotional problem.

To achieve these ends the therapist, over a short period of time, must create a therapeutic atmosphere, establish an alliance with the patient, agree with him as to the definition of the problem to be solved, and utilize the patient's positive feelings for him as the main therapeutic tool. He must use anxiety-provoking questions in order to obtain the evidence he needs to substantiate or to modify his formulation. Also, by utilizing confrontations and clarifications, he must stimulate the patient to examine the areas of emotional difficulty which he tends to avoid in order to help him become aware of his feelings, experience the conflicts, and learn new ways of solving his problem. If the therapist is successful in his efforts, he achieves the stated goals of this kind of psychotherapy and is confident that the patient will use this novel experience and these newly developed problem-solving techniques to deal with the new critical situations in the future.

A great deal has been written about psychotherapy. There is no lack of good books for anyone interested in the subject. Therefore, no effort will be made to review the different schools of thought, the various theories and techniques, and the voluminous literature on this subject. Rather, because of the many prejudiced views about the scientific worth of psychotherapy, this additional volume, which presents a factual account, as well as a conceptual frame of reference for a specialized psychotherapy of short duration, which can be taught systematically to psychiatry residents and other interested professionals during individual supervisory sessions, may help to clarify some of the misconceptions about it. Although a well-educated psychodynamic psychiatrist is best equipped to evaluate and at times to predict human behavior, very little use has been made of such psychiatrists in such vital areas as the selection of students for a college, or the psychological assessment of those seeking political office.

There is another reason for writing this book. Ever since man recognized the need to know, to learn, and to remain free, and used the Socratic dialogue as his method of instruction, the framework of the dyadic relationship has remained as the best way to study man, and as such it is the cornerstone of psychodynamic psychiatry. Individual psychotherapy capital-izes on the therapist-patient interaction. It uses this dyadic relationship to explore freely the patient's emotional problem in order to help him to understand himself.

In anxiety-provoking psychotherapy, neither is the therapist in the familiar role of the all-knowledgeable and authoritative medical doctor who takes specific actions to alter or cure his patient's illness nor is the individual who is engaged in it in the traditional role of the passive and receiving patient. The psychotherapeutic interaction promises nothing more than a systematic investigation of all the factors which may play a role in producing the patient's emotional difficulties. This task is pursued relentlessly in the search for the truth. The patient understands that whatever he discovers about himself within the context of the psychotherapeutic interaction will not be judged by the therapist. He also knows that he is free to choose — to accept or reject whatever he wishes.

Psychotherapy furthermore is an intensive learning process which offers vast educational opportunities to both the therapist and the patient, who, by the way, may be better labeled teacher and student. In these times of materialism, fragmentation, and indifference, these days when people fail to communicate and when they use double messages full of cliches, it is encouraging that there still exists a humanitarian approach which offers the opportunity both to understand and to learn.

Psychodynamic psychotherapy may be criticized as being expensive, available only to few, and emphasizing the individual too much. All these comments are valid. In my opinion, however, every man is entitled to the luxury of an approach, however costly, which is designed to study him in detail. It is because his mind is so complicated that he deserves to have a thorough effort made to understand him in depth. For, despite his biological primate background, despite his tragic ability to destroy, despite his catastrophic capacity to multiply, which may ruin him in the end, man is unique and complex and without any doubt he is, and will always be, "the measure of all things."

Finally, there is a problem with the way in which one presents the subject matter of psychotherapy itself. Should he emphasize the artistic or the scientific point of view? If he stresses the former, he may be criticized as being unscientific, while if he deals only with the latter, he may be accused of having denuded psychotherapy from its vitality and spontaneity and of having portrayed the doctor-patient relationship as a dull and lifeless interaction. I have tried to walk through "the strait gate and narrow way," but here and there I may have stumbled.

The psychotherapeutic work which will be described in the ensuing chapters was conducted in the Psychiatry Clinic of the Massachusetts General Hospital, while I was its director, from May 1954 to July 1968. During this time the clinic population was composed largely of self-referred, relatively well-educated young people who gave freely of their time and were eager to help in whatever way they could with our efforts to evaluate the outcome of short-term anxiety-provoking psychotherapy.

Although the individuals we treated represented only a small part of the great numbers of patients who needed psychiatric help, the group may have been large enough to demonstrate the struggles to be free from rigid attitudes, and to witness the joy of successes. I am grateful to them for giving me a chance

> To see a world in a grain of sand
> And a Heaven in a wild flower,
> Hold infinity in the palm of a hand
> And Eternity in an hour[1]

I want to take this opportunity, therefore, to thank them for their cooperation and to reassure them that sufficient changes have been made in this book to protect confidentiality without any basic alteration of the truth.

Special mention is also due to Drs. Robert Cserr, Donald Fern, Miguel Leibovich, and Mr. Steven Lorch for evaluating and treating several of the patients in our research study.

I wish to express my gratitude to my friend, Dr. Fred Frankel, for his special attention to detail and for his innumerable helpful suggestions pertaining to this manuscript.

I want to thank Dr. Howard Blane for his help with statistics and the research methods which were used and Drs. Randolph Catlin and Edward Messner, who for many years acted as evaluators of patients before and after psychotherapy.

Valuable suggestions and comments about the manuscript were made by Drs. Jarl Jorstad, Cavin Leeman, Paul Russell, and Miss Ruth Westheimer, and credit is due to Miss Dorothy Clark for her perseverance in getting in touch with elusive patients and for making the complicated arrangements for the follow-up interviews.

For editing my manuscript in her meticulous way I am grateful to Cora F. Holbrook, and to my secretaries, who deciphered my handwriting and retyped innumerable copies of this book, I want to express my admiration and appreciation. I am grateful to my daughter Nan for proofreading this book.

To Dr. David Malan, whose pioneering research work in brief psychotherapy has inspired me, and whose ideas, suggestions, and criticisms have stimulated me to seek his advice repeatedly in the pleasant atmosphere of London, I want to express grateful thanks.

Without the relentless and stimulating questioning about theoretical, clinical, and research issues of Dr. Michael McGuire, whose sense of humor made our discussions exciting and our disagreements enjoyable, this book would not have been possible. I express my deep gratitude to him.

I am indebted to my friend, Dr. John C. Nemiah, for his kindness in writing the foreword, and for his continued support and encouragement during his tenure as Acting Chief of Psychiatry of the Massachusetts General Hospital, and particular, as Chief of the Psychiatry Service of the Beth Israel Hospital, for creating an academic atmosphere where relaxed discussions can take place and time can be found for me to write.

Finally, the memory of the late Dr. George Talland comes to mind. His rigorous but constructive criticisms about psychotherapy, his open-minded willingness to treat patients under supervision, his genuine scientific interest in setting up performance tests to assess results, his ready eagerness to discuss history, literature, and art will never be forgotten.

Several reports of our work were first published in various journals and will be acknowledged specifically. I do want, however, to express my special thanks to the editors of *The American Journal of Psychiatry*, *Mental Hygiene*, and *The*

Psychiatric Quarterly for giving me permission to report parts of their content in detail.

It should be stated at this point that I shall not attempt in this book to present a scientific or statistical validation of our findings nor to offer an explanation of the operative therapeutic factors. Beyond a doubt, my technique will be criticized and my theory disputed, the research methods will be challenged, and the results questioned. Nevertheless, I shall present our observations to satisfy the curiosity of my readers, and in the hope that they may prove stimulating to residents in psychiatry, social workers, medical students, and other young people in allied disciplines who are eager to witness the psychological process as a continuum and who like to see the endless variations in pattern and style offered to them by patients while they try to explore the magnificent horizons of their minds.

I also hope that physicians, psychiatrists, and all those who have an interest in psychotherapy will experience, when they read the case material, almost the same fascination as the author felt when he was treating his patients.

Peter E. Sifneos, M.D.
January 1971

CONTENTS

Introduction   1

Part I: Conceptual Frame of Reference   9

1: The First Patient: A Historical Perspective   11
2: Psychological Process as a Dynamic Continuum   22
3: A Concept of Emotional Crisis   29
4: Two Different Kinds of Psychotherapy of Short Duration   44
5: Anxiety-Provoking Psychotherapy, Crisis Intervention   57

Part II: Technical Aspects   73

6: Selection of Patients   75
7: Technique   93
8: Results   124

Part III: Case Reports   145

9: Anxiety, Frigidity, and Agoraphobia   147
10: Anxiety and Homosexuality   169
11: Anxiety and Examination Phobia   194
12: Anxiety and Heterosexual Difficulties   214

SHORT-TERM PSYCHOTHERAPY AND EMOTIONAL CRISIS

INTRODUCTION

Psychotherapy Beleaguered?

Certain aspects of psychiatric classification, of the relations of psychiatry to science in general and medicine in particular, of the field of psychodynamics, and finally of community mental health, should be mentioned briefly at the outset because they tend to complicate any discussion of the subject of psychotherapy.[1] During the nineteenth century, while medicine was able to create a microscopic pathological basis for disease processes and developed effective regimens for treating them, psychiatry was unable either to establish clear-cut pathological criteria for mental illnesses or to set up specific treatment modalities other than custodial care. Frustrated by this failure, psychiatrists continued the search for specific cerebral lesions in order to make their diagnosis; but, except for a few diseases, such as general paresis, they were essentially unsuccessful. Yet no microscopic pathology was discovered to underlie the majority of psychiatric illnesses, and despite the efforts to collect and group together clinical observations and to set up psychiatric syndromes based on the presenting symptoms, no general agreement was reached as to either the label or the language that should be used. The resulting classifications were of little value for communication between psychiatrists.

Because of the difficulties of symptom classification, a

1

different approach became necessary. Freud's understanding of human behavior from a psychodynamic point of view implied that the psychological processes responsible for the production of symptoms, rather than the symptoms themselves, could be studied advantageously. Static nosologies could be abandoned and replaced by this fluid and dynamic method. Wide horizons were opened.

More recently, although the contributions from basic sciences such as neurophysiology, neurochemistry, and neuropharmacology, and the developments in genetics, social sciences, public health, and existential philosophy have enlarged the scope of psychiatry, they have at the same time complicated the relationship of psychiatry with other fields of medicine because of psychiatry's failure to establish a scientific foundation. Furthermore, because the subject matter of psychiatry deals with elusive changes rather than with verifiable concreteness it has been criticized as being vague and superficial. Irony and ridicule have, at times, marked this controversy. Do psychiatrists have any "hard facts" to teach? Is psychiatric treatment any good, we are asked, or is it all a matter of common sense? The inevitable conclusion is reached that although psychiatry must be tolerated, it should be relegated to the position of a second-rate specialty.

In response to this pomposity about science, as presented by some who were "more royalist than the king," and who usually were internists or surgeons, some psychiatrists became apologetic about their specialty, while others, fearful and apathetic, withdrew from their medical colleagues, surrounded themselves with jargon, and isolated themselves behind the protection of their private practice. These polemical discussions have created problems, which are exemplified by the present state of psychosomatic medicine, where most often either biological or psychological factors are emphasized and rarely the interrelations of both.[1]

Despite these outer differences, the contact between psychiatry and medicine has been of some limited value to both. The existence of psychiatric wards in general hospitals and psychiatrists called as consultants by their medical colleagues, have forced an awareness of the importance of the psychological understanding of patients. Furthermore, psychiatric departments borrowing from the experiences of medical education and public health, have focused on the study of psychological phenomena in both mentally ill and mentally healthy individuals and have tried to teach psychiatric residents how to take the necessary steps for the development of preventive measures against mental illness.

There is another factor, however, which may bring medicine and psychiatry closer together. This involves the swift advances and contributions from the basic sciences which are rapidly making microscopic pathology obsolete as an overall basis for medicine. This necessitates the establishment of a new biochemical pathology which will require thorough knowledge in the future of each patient's individual biochemistry. Faced with this situation, medicine will be confronted with similar problems, which, at the present time, are encountered by the psychiatrist, who must understand the infinitesimally complex psychological processes of each individual patient.

Paradoxical as it may seem at first to compare biochemistry to psychodynamic psychiatry and to imply that they have something in common, this is indeed the case. Both deal with dynamic processes and utilize the same analytic or synthetic methods of inquiry. In this context, therefore, both biochemistry or psychodynamic psychiatry are inexorably committed to a continuous pursuit of uncertainty, of understanding, and of change, which is truly scientific. Although every function of the brain can ultimately be reduced to intricate chemical reactions, there is no doubt that because of the different genetic and environmental background surrounding each individual, chemically or psychologically every man will differ from every other man. In the final analysis, therefore, although the functions of the brain will be qualitatively and quantitatively chemical, they will have to be studied and understood idiosyncratically.

This discussion may be academic just now because, at present, the psychological processes cannot be either presented or explained in biochemical terms. Psychodynamics, on the other hand, emphasize the qualitative and quantitative differences between individuals, and although they require greater skills, different ways of observing, and different techniques of interviewing, they offer enormous advantages because they open up vast possibilities of understanding the human mind.

The study of the conscious and unconscious interactions between conflicts, drives, feelings, fantasies, and thoughts offers us new opportunity but also presents us with a problem which, at first glance, appears to be insoluble. The psychiatrist, however (who learns to view each emotional difficulty of his patients as being the result of a continuous psychological process, differing only in style and pattern, which must be understood in order to help him overcome it) is best prepared, in my opinion, to resolve this problem and to understand his fellow man. Psychodynamics then must become the basis of all psychotherapy.

There are dangers implicit in the psychodynamic approach. Unconscious motivations which had been hidden, covered up, and rationalized give rise to enormous resistance when they are interfered with, and hostility against the therapist starts to rise. These theoretical considerations, furthermore, should not obscure certain current realities. For 2500 years man has been confronted with the classical dilemma between individual freedom and social conformity. The old controversy over the role of the university coupled with the recent campus riots has highlighted this conflict. Academic psychiatry also has been torn between continuing to place its traditional emphasis on painstakingly thorough psychodynamic understanding of the individual and trying to solve social problems. It must decide whether to stay in the university and its teaching hospital or to establish itself in the community.

Confronted by a rise in world population, shortages of psychiatrists, increased psychological sophistication of the public, relentless demands and unrealistic expectations for increased services, psychiatry must start looking for answers. In a world where distances become shorter and shorter, when real communication between people becomes progressively poorer and poorer, when vital decisions as to our very survival rest in the hands of fewer and fewer people, when the pressures on psychiatrists to become involved in social and political issues and to abandon their traditional interests becomes stronger and stronger, obviously a balance must be achieved.

This has not occurred, however. The concept of community mental health with its emphasis on populations rather than on the individual is riding a crest of popularity; mental health professionals, though many are poorly trained, are offered well-paying positions. Furthermore, they are viewed by the public as possessing unusual powers and offering the promise of unending happiness. The stereotyped public image of the psychiatrist is already distorted. He is viewed either as an omnipotent individual whose magical powers can solve all problems or as an eccentric to be ridiculed or feared. Such tarnished and exaggerated views reinforce the overall confusion. Despite this fact, the demands for public services to bring about this happy illusion continue. The mental health professionals, instead of attempting to define the limitations of community mental health, have encouraged these magical expectations by promises of abundant services, while they have made little effort to find out what services are needed and how they can be implemented. Sooner or later these expectations of the public will explode into increasing demands for a tangible evidence of the value of these promises. Reality will catch up with the fantasy, and there will be many disappointments.

The argument has been advanced that psychotherapy takes too long, that it is expensive in time and money, and that it is aimed toward only a few people with middle- or upper-class values. Psychotherapy has been a victim of these attitudes, and it has been dismissed easily as being old fashioned, to be replaced by vaguely defined "better services." The question which must be raised and answered realistically at this point is: "What does psychotherapy have to offer?" Prevailing opinions about this differ. From one extreme — because of the subjective reports of enthusiastic patients and their therapists — it is presented as a panacea for all emotional ills.

On the other hand, because of the criticisms already enumerated and because, with few exceptions, very little effort has been made to present convincing evidence of a successful result to the objective outside observer, the impression has been created that it is unscientific and, by and large, ineffective. In general, many of the difficulties encountered in trying to evaluate the results of psychotherapy have given rise to inertia and have discouraged the majority of psychiatrists. This book, then, will attempt to give a factual and detailed account of short-term anxiety-provoking psychotherapy and its outcome.

It opens with the case presentation of the first patient we treated with this kind of short-term psychotherapy. Apart from its historical significance, much was learned from that psychotherapeutic relationship. We profited greatly from our mistakes.

The "psychological process," which is viewed as a dynamic continuum, and the "emotional crisis" which is considered as a focal point as well as a turning point along this continuum, are the subjects of the following two chapters. In Chapter 4 a conceptual frame of reference is developed for two kinds of psychotherapy of short duration. Chapter 5 deals with anxiety-provoking psychotherapy in general and crisis intervention in particular. Short-term anxiety-provoking psychotherapy is discussed in Part II. The evaluation and selection of patients according to a set of specific criteria, the requirements for this type of psychotherapy, and the technique used are presented systematically. A discussion of the results of this kind of treatment concludes this section of the book. The third part deals with the clinical material. Three case examples, followed by a more detailed presentation of fifteen interviews with a patient, are used to demonstrate, as explicitly as possible, the technique of short-term anxiety-provoking psychotherapy.

My notes had to be edited, of course, so as to keep the anonymity of the patients and the confidentiality of their communications. These changes, however, do not alter the basic observations, nor do they influence the presentation of the psychotherapeutic process. I have tried to maintain the continuity of the interviews and to keep intact the spontaneity of the doctor-patient interaction, with as few interruptions as possible. On occasion, however, certain technical clarifications and comments have been inserted for the benefit of the unsophisticated. I appeal for the indulgence of those readers to whom all this is obvious.

I hope that by presenting the case material extensively enough, and sufficiently in detail, I shall provide the reader with the evidence he needs to assess and to answer for himself the questions about the efficacy and the results of this kind of short-term psychotherapy. I also hope that by presenting the criteria for evaluation necessary for the selection of patients systematically, even if they have been arrived at empirically, and the technical requirements explicitly, I shall convince the educators that it is possible to structure the teaching of psychotherapy. Above and beyond these considerations, however, I hope to demonstrate to students that it is possible to learn to use short-term anxiety-provoking psychotherapy effectively.

Part I. A CONCEPTUAL FRAME OF REFERENCE

1

THE FIRST PATIENT: A HISTORICAL PERSPECTIVE

A twenty-eight-year-old single white male student came to the Psychiatry Clinic of the Massachusetts General Hospital complaining of nervousness which he associated with his decision to be married in two months' time.[1] The thought of being looked at as the center of attention by many people during the wedding ceremony caused him to become tense. He was particularly conscious of this nervousness when he was riding the subway, which frightened him so much that he had to walk to school. He also experienced a recurrence of fear of buses, trains, cars, and enclosures of all sorts which had manifested itself periodically during his childhood. He had a variety of physical symptoms, such as stomach pains, a sensation of "trembling inside," difficulty in breathing, occasional diarrhea, attacks of perspiration, and generalized weakness. As a result of all this he became irritable with his fiancée and with people at school. His main reason for coming to the clinic was a request for help to overcome his fear of the marriage ceremony.

He dated his present illness to a "panic spell" which he experienced while serving in the army two years prior to his coming to the clinic. On that occasion, while he was standing at attention during a command performance he became apprehensive and faint. When his commanding officer approached, he felt weak at the thought of being "looked over," suddenly everything "went black," and he fainted. Soon after this episode he was honorably discharged from the army.

When he returned to Boston he slowly developed a fear of buses and subway trains; he also remembered being afraid of high places and elevators and said he had experienced shortness of breath dating to the age of ten. Three months before coming to the clinic he met a girl with whom he fell in love. They soon became engaged and started to make plans for their wedding in a Catholic ceremony. As their arrangements crystallized, he noticed that his phobias were progressively intensified. He was also, at times, afraid of hoodlums or "crazy people" who might jump on him from behind. Finally, he went to talk with a priest about his condition. He felt dissatisfied after their conversation, and it was at this point that he came to the clinic for help.

The patient was the younger of two children. His brother was five years older than he. His father, whom he described as kind but also temperamental, had died when he was four years old. One episode which stood out in his memory had to do with striking his head and bleeding while his father comforted and loved him. Visibly tremulous, he recalled his father as sick in a bed and barely able to breathe. He said he did not cry after his father died; on the contrary, he remembered with joy his trip to New York with his mother and brother after his father's funeral. Yet at the same time he had a train phobia. When the family returned to Boston a few months later, his mother had to go to work to support the children. He was frightened whenever his mother left the house, but he said his brother always took good care of him.

He described his mother as strong and domineering. She was still living and well at sixty-eight, had remarried when the patient was eight years old, and completely dominated her second husband. The family finances improved greatly, but his mother continued to work and kept all the money she earned for herself.

The patient was a good student and had many friends of both sexes. He considered himself a leader and described himself as "the life of the party" at social gatherings; but, as he grew older, he became more and more apprehensive socially. He relied for reassurance on people who liked him because he considered himself a coward. He said he always had "a funny nervous feeling inside," which he could not explain. At the age of eighteen, after graduation from high school with honors, he got a job. As a result he felt much more secure and financially independent, and, as a result of this, he decided to leave the Catholic Church. This major decision gave rise to a conflict. He was frightened at times, while, on other occasions, he felt independent and in no need "to lean on anything or anyone."

At twenty-six he was drafted into the army, and it was during this time that he had his first sexual experience, which was with a prostitute. He said he was impotent but rationalized it by blaming it on his having been drunk at the time. It appeared that this episode had occurred one week before the army inspection when he fainted.

Upon returning to Boston he dated a great many girls, and it was at this time that his physical symptoms and his bus and subway fears slowly started to reappear. Despite these symptoms, he became engaged to his "steady" girl friend, and when she invited him to live with her he accepted. For about six months they were fairly happy and had satisfactory sexual relations. Soon after, he met an older woman with whom he started to have sexual intercourse. This led to his breaking up with his steady girl friend, "because of incompatibilities in our personalities," he said. Three months before coming to the clinic he met his future wife, and immediately he fell in love with her. Soon they were engaged and were making active plans for their wedding. It was after they decided to have a Catholic ceremony that his phobias and other physical symptoms became intensified and eventually led to his coming to the psychiatry clinic for help.

When asked to describe his relationship with his brother, he smiled and dismissed him as "a professional man, married, with two children, who is otherwise a very boring person." They rarely saw each other now, nor did he visit his mother very often. He was working in a bookstore at night and going to college during the day. He had several close male friends. He was a hard worker, and his academic record was excellent.

His medical history was essentially negative, and a report from his family physician showed that he was in good health. His physical examination, laboratory tests, and X-rays were all within normal limits.

The patient was fairly tall and neatly dressed. His facial expression was somewhat anxious. He related well with the interviewer but tended to be a bit ingratiating. Toward the end of the interview, looking tense and perspiring profusely, he asked, "Well, Doctor, we have talked for quite some time but you haven't answered my question. Can you help me get married by the fifteenth of November?"

Let us stop here for a moment.

When this patient was presented at grand rounds of the psychiatric staff of the Massachusetts General Hospital this same question was raised. Here are the kinds of questions which were asked about the patient's psychological makeup: What were his strengths? What about his transient impotence? What was the significance of his decision to leave the Catholic Church as well as to decide later to be married there? What techniques should be used to deal with his phobias on a short-term basis? What personality changes could one expect over a brief period of time? What would happen to his somewhat passive-dependent features? What about his relation with his brother and his mother?

The staff were required to answer some of their own questions. It was considered that if the initial assessment of the patient's strength was correct, it could be expected that the prognosis was good for meeting the deadline. It was thought that if a good relationship could be established with the patient which would encourage him to trust his doctor, this would give him the confidence that a description of all his feelings would be considered acceptable to the therapist. This, in turn, could improve his self-esteem. It was also hoped that his symptoms could be altered significantly to help him feel better and develop freer relationships with people.

Many more questions can be raised. What is this patient's

basic emotional problem? What are the significant psychological conflicts underlying his difficulties? What is the significance of the predisposing factors and of the specific and stressful events which precipitated his emotional crisis? What are his psychodynamics? What are his true interpersonal relations? What connection is there between the phobias he presented and his physical symptoms? What is his relationship with his fiancée and with women in general? What psychotherapeutic techniques should we utilize in treating him? Should we reassure him, give him drugs, or even electric shock treatment? What results should we aim to obtain? What symptomatic relief can we expect? What help can we offer him which would enable him to define, and possibly learn to solve, his problem, and thereby utilize what he will have learned during the treatment in solving new problems which may arise in his life? What criteria can we establish for the selection of other patients with similar problems? These are some of the questions that arose in my mind in August 1956.

Let us now return to our patient. He was accepted for psychotherapy because his challenging questions about helping him to get married and the imminent deadline date which he gave aroused my interest. I therefore decided to proceed with his treatment, which started in October of that year. There were exactly seven weeks left to the date of his wedding.

In the first interview he had announced that he walked to the hospital because he was afraid to take the subway. He looked tense and dejected, and asked for a "pill" to help him calm down. I refused to grant his request, saying that we should try to understand what made him feel tense rather than trying to eliminate his tension right away. He was annoyed by this remark, but he seemed to accept it. He mentioned that he had always been afraid of people "jumping on him." He said that he did not like to fight because he was afraid "of being hurt," which made him feel like a coward; but that occasionally he felt strong and powerful and at these times he considered himself able to fight anyone anywhere. As an example of this attitude, he said that when he was eighteen years old he had a good job, felt strong and independent, and, being in this mood, he had decided to abandon the Catholic Church. This decision surprised him because he was very religious and had always been dependent on the church for its "protective influence." "By confessing, all is forgiven," he exclaimed significantly, and winked. When I asked him what he meant by this, he announced that he knew a priest who liked him and whom he felt he could manipulate. He said this with a smile; but then he became serious and added that all this had changed. "Now I am full of fears. Bridges make me nervous. So do tall places and tunnels. I also have trouble with my boss at work. It's the same thing all over again, as it was when I was in the army. I have the strange feeling that my boss does not like me." I pointed out that this was a different situation from the one in which he had manipulated the priest. He smiled again and said that this had occurred to him because both his commanding officer and his boss were very nice, yet recently he had felt quite apprehensive and he had not dared to ask his boss for an increase in his pay.

These associations made him remember a time when he was alone in the house with his brother. His mother had gone to work, and he was playing in the kitchen with his toy guns when he realized that his brother was not in the house. He looked everywhere but was unable to find him. He soon became very alarmed and rushed out of the house. As he ran down the street he saw his mother and brother walking together toward the house. They saw him and waved, but he felt intensely jealous; and turning away, he walked back home alone, wiping the tears from his eyes. He was unable to explain in what way the jealousy of his brother was associated with his difficulty with his boss or the commanding officer.

He arrived twenty minutes early for his second interview, saying that he had felt nervous about a premarital blood test but was able to take it. He appeared to be very tense. He talked at length about his teachers at school and about how every student in speech class had to give a talk in front of an audience, and how frightened he felt with all the students looking at him. "At such times I get shortness of breath and a 'trembling feeling' inside. My heart starts to pound, and I think I am dying." He said this shortness of breath always reminded him of being breathless, which made him feel guilty because it was associated with his masturbating when he was twelve years old. He remembered that on one occasion his brother, who had noticed his breathlessness, had commented that this was a sign of serious sickness and that he might die. This frightened him, and he felt very angry because he thought his brother said it on purpose in order to laugh at him. During this interview he tried to emphasize how weak he felt and how much he was in need of pills; but I emphasized that I was not impressed by his requests because I was convinced that he was able to understand the reasons for these feelings.

In the third interview he said that he had skipped class. He emphasized that he was incapable of going through the torture of having to give a lecture in front of the group. He came early to the hospital and walked up and down the corridors, looking forward to his three o'clock appointment with me. When he was asked what precipitated this running away from his responsibilities, he paused for a while and then he mentioned having gone to the movies with his fiancée the previous night. It was a murder picture. Finally the murderer was caught and was about to be electrocuted. It was at this point that he became panicky and ran out before the end of the show. While smoking a cigarette in the lobby, he started to tremble and developed shortness of breath. He said he was afraid that he was making a spectacle of himself but felt reassured when his fiancée put her arms around him. He then turned to me and asked, "Are you going to cut the interview short today?" This thought had flashed into his mind when he was telling me about the murderer who was to be electrocuted. I asked him to tell me more about this fear, and he talked about having always been terrified of razors, knives, and of going to the barber shop. He added that he had never been shaved by a barber because "the razor comes too close and those sharp edges really make me shudder." He said that he always went to a barber who used an electric shaver, who was sympathetic and understood his phobias. I explained to him that he was taking the easy way out, and I emphasized that these feelings were also associated with the fear of my "cutting" him by an early termination of the interview. I encouraged him to discuss the way he felt about me. He looked puzzled at first and then replied that he had suddenly remembered an episode that happened when he was eight years old. It was at the time when his stepfather had left to go to war, and he was sleeping in the same room with his brother. "Before leaving, my stepfather had told me that after he was gone I was going to be 'the man of the house.' I recall having shortness of breath that night and I could not sleep." He said that he sat up in bed and cried. He asked himself queer questions, such as "Is my heart beating?" "Am I breathing?" "Am I dead?" Then the frightening thought occurred to him. "If I die I will be put in a black, closed place. I was paralyzed with fears. I called my mother and asked her if I was breathing. My brother was fed up with me, and my mother got quite upset and told me that I could sleep in my stepfather's bed next to her own." This was the bed in which his father had died after suffering a heart attack and having what appeared to have been pulmonary edema terminally. When I asked him to tell me more about this he said he remembered his father as sitting up in bed, unable to breathe. This picture had remained fixed in his mind. "Now I was in my father's bed," he said, "but the funny thing about it was that my shortness of breath went away." His mother let him sleep with her for a while, and he remembered masturbating and having fantasies about intercourse with women who were much older than he. He then remembered that when he was four years old he had been caught naked by his father in a closet with a little girl, but he did not remember having been punished at that time. I tried to connect this episode with the patient's fear of subways and buses, but he was unimpressed by that suggestion. "Maybe there is something to it, Doc," was his only comment, which shattered my efforts.

In the fourth hour he told me that he had given "his speech" despite his terror. He said that as soon as he started to talk, he realized that everything was going to be all right. He did a creditable job and was congratulated by his teachers and the other students. He felt very proud. He then changed the subject.

"This closet business we talked about last time reminds me of the train ride to New York after my father died. I have been doing some thinking, trying to figure out what had happened, and it was then that I remembered. We were waiting for the train, and when I finally saw it approach, the big engine 'puffing' as if it couldn't breathe, I was scared. When I saw it coming at me I thought it was going to jump the track and get me. I was terrified. Maybe all this had something to do with being caught in that closet with the girl." I reminded him of my unsuccessful attempts to connect these two episodes. He smiled and said that he felt he had to do all the work for himself. I agreed, and again I tried to underscore the connection between his present-day phobias, the closet episode, his father's death, and the recent memory about the train engine. He looked amazed after this obvious clarification, which I thought he had already made for himself, and added, "I never realized that my father was going to punish me for that business in the closet. Because he never did so, I have been scared that he was going to do it after he died."

In the fifth interview he announced that he felt much better. He talked about all the thinking he had done during the week and recounted the details of a tonsillectomy when he was four. He also talked about the feeling of being attacked or of attacking others. When I asked him to tell me more about all this he said that nobody had ever attacked him, because he was always considered to be "tough." "I am scared of that vicious feeling inside me. When you get into a fight and you get mad, you may kill someone, and I'll get the electric chair." I did not have to remind him of the recent feeling he had experienced at the movies. He sighed and associated this fear with having been told by his mother that people become insane or die when they are vicious, or do bad things, such as masturbate as his brother had suggested; but then he proceeded to describe with considerable pride an incident in Korea when he had to fight two men who were trying to attack a girl. He was smiling broadly when he departed.

During the sixth and last interview before the wedding he said that many of his fears had decreased but that the subway phobia still persisted. He said that he could see a connection between the fear of loss of his manhood and his interest in "bad sexual practices" which had led to fear of punishment and the feeling of being a coward. When asked about this further, he said that he was still apprehensive about the wedding ceremony but that he had decided he was going to go through with it anyway. He told himself that it was not going to be as bad as he had expected. He again brought up the shortness of breath, the fear of death, and his tonsillectomy. Then he suddenly became visibly pale and announced that something new had suddenly popped into his mind, and he went on: "The day my stepfather returned from the war, I had an appendectomy. I was twelve years old. It was nearing Christmas time. I missed my mother while in the hospital and I was angry with her and with my stepfather for keeping her away from me. After my stepfather told me that I was going to be the 'man of the house' I was sure that I was never going to see him again. It was going to be like my real father. He would also die. I wished that he would never come back, but he did. I remember, in the hospital, having that shortness of breath and the fear that I was going to die whenever I thought of my mother and my stepfather together." And then, as if on second thought, he added, "It was also the fear of what he would do to me. The same feeling like the razor at the barber shop — too close, too sharp. Things are cut off, you lose your manhood. I guess you have to be a coward so that these terrible things should not happen to you."

I saw him three weeks later. All had gone according to schedule at his wedding. He said that he was scared before going to the church, but once the ceremony had started he felt that he was the center of attention — everybody was looking at him. It was like giving a speech. Everyone was admiring him. He went to New York by train for his honeymoon, felt a little apprehensive, but managed quite well. He said that while in New York he took the subways regularly to test himself; and then he added significantly, "You know, Doctor, those New York subways are quite something compared to those puny ones we got here in Boston."

I saw him twice more in follow-up. His phobias and physical symptoms had disappeared six months after the treatment was terminated. Two years later during Christmas week all his symptoms suddenly returned. He called for an appointment and was seen the next day but by then he was able to figure out that his fears had recurred exactly six months to the date after his mother had died. He said it was an "anniversary neurosis." After this, he was again asymptomatic.

I came to the conclusion that this man was helped to face the unpleasant emotional conflicts underlying his symptoms. As a result of this and under the special conditions of the transference relation, it was thought by the psychiatric staff that a dynamic change had taken place which consisted of a substitution of the defense mechanisms isolation, displacement, and projection with a counterphobic defense which mastered his anxiety. This resulted in the change of his phobias as well as his physical symptoms. Stopping treatment at that time was forced by the deadline. That one could try to deliberately stop early after this limited amount of work was something that should be looked into. Although the patient's character was not altered fundamentally, it was thought that changes which occurred over such a short period of time should be assessed more systematically because they seemed more or less to have helped the patient overcome his difficulties. If the dynamic changes observed permitted this patient to get through a critical period in his life, such changes in attitude may be lasting and may be an adequate goal of psychotherapy. The implications were clear. They were ripe for exploration and investigation.

2

PSYCHOLOGICAL PROCESSES
AS A DYNAMIC CONTINUUM

The Question Is How Much?

The difficulties of psychiatric nosology are complicated by the perennial controversy over the role played by genetic factors versus the role played by the environment. This has tended to present a fragmented picture of psychiatric illness. From studies of identical twins, it appears that genetic factors play an important part in the development of schizophrenia. It has been advocated by Pauling[1] that orthomolecular psychiatry may control mental illness by varying the concentration of substances normally present in the human body and maintaining an optimum molecular composition of the brain. The search for chemical substances as the causes of schizophrenia also continues unabated.[2] It was suggested recently that an extra Y chromosome leads to aggressive behavior in some individuals. Finally, certain well-documented studies point to the limbic system as playing an important role in emotions and as leading to overwhelming aggressive behavior when certain parts of the limbic system are artificially stimulated or pathologically damaged. On the other hand, studies on child development emphasize the role of social and cultural disturbances in the family. Experimental isolation of laboratory-reared rhesus monkeys gives rise to persistent abnormal behavior[3] Instrumental learning produces modifications in such physiological responses as heart rate, blood pressure, intestinal contraction, and formation of the urine in the kidney,[4] to mention only a few. All these investigations point to the important role played by the environment.

Although such studies are very interesting in themselves, their immediate relevance is still remote to our understanding of the psychological process which confronts us as clinicians. Consider the following illustrative cases:

CASE 1. A thirty-five-year-old advertising salesman wants to get a big corporation contract for his firm. He has heard that the key to this achievement lies with the vice-president of that company. He makes a systematic investigation of this executive and finds out that one of the things he enjoys most is a good meal in a French restaurant. He prepares his plan of action. He invites the executive to such a restaurant, orders Le Montrachet 1964 to be served with the lobster, and Le Chambertin 1961 for the steak; and, after dinner, having created a pleasant atmosphere over coffee, cognac, and good cigars, he is able to persuade the guest to place an order with his firm.

CASE 2. A twenty-year-old girl is engaged to be married.[5] Her fiancé decides to postpone the wedding for six months. She is very angry, and they quarrel, but she finally acquiesces, warning him, however, not to postpone the marriage again, and adding, significantly, "because otherwise you'll be sorry." Six months later, the wedding having been formally announced, her fiancé asks for one month's postponement because the opportunity has arisen for him to earn a thousand dollars, which he could use as a down payment for their new house. The girl is angry, a tirade ensues, and she finally threatens him with, "If you do not reconsider you will be sorry." When he asks her what she means by this threat, she implies vaguely that she might try to kill herself. The argument continues, threats and counterthreats are exchanged. The young girl again repeats her determination to try to kill herself, to which her fiancé angrily retorts, as he is departing, "If you're so foolish, go ahead." With tears in her eyes, she immediately runs to the medicine closet and starts to swallow an assortment of medications belonging to her grandmother. She then proceeds to tell her grandmother what she has done. The old lady, alarmed, calls for an ambulance, notifies the fiancé of what has happened, and asks him to meet them at the emergency ward of the nearest hospital. There a dramatic scene ensues.

The patient is somewhat drowsy, having had her stomach lavaged. Her grandmother is holding her hand, and a nurse makes reassuring noises. At this point the fiancé appears on the scene. At the sight of him the young girl starts lifting a tremulous hand, finally points a finger accusingly at him, and says, "I did it because of you." At this point he also starts to tremble, asks for forgiveness, and promises not to interfere again with the wedding plans. A faint smile is then detected on the young woman's face. After a good night's sleep she is cheerful and asks to be discharged from the ward where she was admitted. When questioned about her paradoxical behavior after having attempted to kill herself the night before, she smiles and says, "But things have changed drastically. We are still going to be married on the day I have announced." Her fiancé, still tremulous, also asks that she may be allowed to go home so that they may proceed with their wedding arrangements according to plan. He begged us to discharge his fiancée because her continued hospitalization made him feel guilty.

Both cases involve manipulation. In the first case it is considered only moderate and therefore acceptable, while in the second, it is excessive and therefore pathological. Thus, it is only a matter of degree. The question is how much?

Under ordinary circumstances, an individual may be able to function adequately while tolerating a certain degree of anxiety. The amount of anxiety which may be considered pathological is a question to be raised. Since we have no specific measurement for these quantitative differences at the present time, and since there are no clear-cut lines of demarcation between mental health and mental illness, we must try to understand both the quantitative and the qualitative aspects of every individual emotional problem as a psychodynamic continuum of psychological processes which differ only in degree.

The following example may illustrate this point: A man is hurrying to get a plane which will take him to an important business appointment in another city. While he is driving his car faster and faster he is forced to stop at a red light. At the next intersection, he has to stop again. This is repeated a third time. Looking at his watch in a state of irritation, he honks his horn at another car which is slow to get started. He races along, but as his car is approaching the fourth intersection, after all the other cars managed to go through, the light turns red. At this point, his annoyance reaches its peak, and the thought that the plane has departed and that he will miss his important business contract looms as serious in his mind. Frustrated, he mumbles angrily, "The world is against me today." Such an irritating episode, however, is usually easily forgotten. Even if our businessman continues to think about it for a few hours or a day or two and recounts it to his wife or his friends, it is still considered to be within normal limits. On the other hand, if he is unable to forget it, is preoccupied with it for a week or more, talks incessantly to everybody about it, and has difficulty in sleeping — such behavior is considered to be mildly neurotic. A patient who seems to be unable to forget an annoyance, who becomes depressed, who constantly and repetitively thinks that everything is against him, who slowly becomes unable to function, and who finally is suspicious of everybody — such a patient could be called paranoid and may have to be admitted to a mental hospital.

Psychiatric facilities in various countries of the world may differ in the way in which they would deal with such problems. Neurotic, or even mild, emotional problems may be considered acceptable for treatment in the United States or Norway, while the majority of India's psychiatric facilities deal only with severely disturbed or with psychotic patients. In addition, social and cultural differences complicate the psychological evaluation of the patient. The aberrations which one society may tolerate as normal and another consider as eccentric is, at times, intriguing to observe. An anthropologist friend of mine related how a Central American Indian village dealt with a schizophrenic man who started to hallucinate. He was immediately elevated to a high social position, and soon became the center of attention of the whole village. It was considered an honor to be close to him and to touch him. He was viewed as a special person, because he could hear the voice of God. This primitive society not only did not consider him sick but raised him to a high status instead of placing him behind "locked doors," as is customary in our "civilized" society!

Another complication may arise when the rules of social behavior are suddenly altered and a behavior which was previously considered unacceptable suddenly becomes the custom of the day. The following account of an ex-soldier speaks for itself:

I was brought up to think of other people. My parents did not believe in violence. I remember, as a little boy, that I was locked up in my room for twenty-four hours because I hit another boy. Another time I was severely punished by my parents for having accidentally killed a puppy. My father spanked me, and my mother did not speak to me for days. From then on I never laid my hands on anyone else. I was unhappy in my childhood. When I eighteen I joined the military service. I had hoped to earn enough money to go to college. My folks were very poor. Then there was Vietnam. I was glad to go there because I had figured that it was my duty to fight for my country. I had never thought that I would have to kill a human being. Army life in Vietnam was exciting. I used to try to help the old folks who didn't have enough to eat. I used to give food to the poor kids who came around our camp begging. I thought my parents would have been proud of me. It all happened so fast. I was on patrol one day. There was a pebble in my boot and it started to hurt, so I stopped to get it out while my buddies moved forward. The next thing I knew all hell broke loose. I saw those guys firing at me. At first, the foolish notion crossed my mind that they were buddies of mine playing some kind of trick on me. I thought it was all a joke. But it was no trick. Blood started to flow all over my sleeve. I felt no pain, but suddenly − I can't describe it − I got so mad I saw red, and then I started to shoot. I knew they were enemy soldiers. My mind went blank. I took aim and I shot at one of them. He fell down, but the others kept on firing. Bullets were whizzing all around. I shot at them, and I could see another one roll over. He screamed with pain. I was glad I hit him. The other two raised their hands, and I knew that they were surrendering, but I had the urge to shoot them, also. Thank God I didn't. I motioned them to stop, to throw down their weapons, and to surrender. I got behind them, and from then on it was easy. I marched them straight down to our lines.

As he was describing all this, he looked almost intoxicated — his mood was elated, and he seemed to enjoy it all. He went on:

The next day I was decorated. After I was discharged I returned home. They gave me a hero's welcome. It was great, but it didn't last. My dad had died while I was away, and my mother couldn't believe what I had done. "Son," she said, "How could you have killed another human being after what I taught you?" She burst into tears. That's all she had to say. I was confused. Soon I had to look around for a job. Most people were nice to me; they all remembered what I had done. Some of the younger kids who used to be my friends tried to avoid me, however. I was offered a job, but I had no training and they wouldn't keep me. I finally got a job in a drugstore, behind the counter. Some of the kids were nice, but some others were downright rude. They were pacifists. Others cared only about their own fun, their cars, and their ball games. I was restless, I was unhappy. I was unable to sleep at night. I didn't care to talk to anybody. I didn't want to go out on dates. Soon the thought came to my mind that I must do away with myself — that there was no hope and no future.

This young man, brought up to believe that killing another person is the worst crime, was forced to change his beliefs overnight. Society had changed the rules of the game. Killing another human being makes one a hero. He is confused when his mother confronts him with what he had done. He finally thinks of suicide as a way out of this impasse. "Civilized" society should congratulate itself for what it has done to this young soldier!

Above and beyond the psychodynamic considerations of this case there is a paradox in the situation. Our soldier-patient is considered to be mentally healthy in the war and mentally ill in peacetime. One would have expected the opposite. Such social situations create difficult problems. What criteria, then, must we use to evaluate this young man? There is no easy answer.

Viewing the psychological processes as a dynamic continuum may give us the best opportunity to understand our suffering patients. To do this we must study the psychodynamics of each individual patient. This involves specialized knowledge, paying particular attention to the endless variations in style and pattern of each patient's emotional problem. One must search for cues in the patient's over-all behavior which may be hidden behind exaggerated postures or distorted facial expressions. He must look for hints in the patient's verbal expression or incongruous reactions in his emotional attitude. He must assess the qualitative differences in the patient's strengths and weaknesses and the major and minor aberrations in his character structure. The capacity to work, the satisfactions and enjoyments, the ability to tolerate anxiety, to face hazards realistically, and to devise new ways to deal with emotional crises — all these must be taken into consideration. Furthermore, emphasis must be placed on the emotional conflicts which underlie the patient's symptoms. One must be aware of all these dimensions while he is scrutinizing the way the patient interacts with other people, for there is no better way to assess a patient's ability to meet the realistic demands of the outside world than by testing his capacity to deal with the fickle inconsistencies of human interactions. This painstaking task is essential in the preparation for the psychotherapeutic work which is to ensue.

Our young ex-soldier was in a state of emotional crisis. In order to understand his psychodynamics we must first evaluate this critical condition. A concept of emotional crisis will be described in the following chapter; it plays a central role in helping us to understand people in distress.

3

A CONCEPT OF EMOTIONAL CRISIS

A Turning Point

An emotional crisis is a focal point in the life-long and ever-changing continuum of psychological processes, and, as such, it gives us a unique opportunity for a cross-sectional study of this longitudinal psychodynamic continuum. The understanding of an emotional crisis throws light on the steps involved in the production of psychiatric symptoms before such symptoms become crystallized into a neurosis; also, it offers the possibility for the preventive actions in the form of psychotherapeutic interventions of short duration required to obviate its development. These psychotherapeutic techniques, which are aimed at helping those individuals who are in the midst of an emotional turmoil, such as "crisis intervention" and "crisis support" will be described briefly in the next two chapters.

An emotional crisis is an "intensification or aggravation of a painful state of being," it is a turning point for better or for worse." Those who seek psychiatric help at times of emotional crisis constitute a small percentage of the millions of people who face hazardous situations and undergo emotional crises — possibly a large enough number to present emotional conflicts, reactions, motivations, and methods used by ordinary human beings at times of stress. It must be remembered, however, that only after an individual has been able to overcome the turbulent disruption of his emotional crisis is he able to return to a mentally healthy level of functioning.

Four case reports illustrate some of these points:

CASE 1. A thirty-five-year-old businessman came to a suburban mental health agency because his wife, after a talk with her minister, had decided to see a psychiatrist. She had been emotionally disturbed for many years, had no friends, was suspicious of people, and drank excessively. She was two years his senior. Her mother, who had been an alcoholic, burned herself to death while drunk. Her father had left the family when she was two years old, and her brother was in prison for theft. This man had met his wife at a bar where she worked as a waitress, was attracted to her, and became excited by the idea of "saving her" from her "terrible life." He asked her to marry him, and she accepted immediately. Despite what he called his wife's "peculiarities," he was always supportive and never antagonized her. For example, he did not complain about her inability to discipline their children nor about her personal carelessness, nor even about the untidy condition of their house. He was understanding of her temper tantrums, even at times when he had to sit up all night listening to tirades of her angry complaints. After a long day's work he cooked the evening meal and then fed, bathed, and put their two children to bed. He derived much satisfaction from all these activities and was proud to be his wife's "savior," "the pillar of support of the whole family." The news of his wife's plan to see a psychiatrist made him realize that his family life could be altered drastically. He was particularly apprenhensive when his wife mentioned that she was optimistic about the psychiatrist's being able to help her. He felt annoyed at the minister who had referred her for psychotherapy. On one occasion when she told him that her psychiatrist was now "her main support," he became anxious and angry. He realized that he was unable to cope with the situation but did not know what to do. When his attempts to persuade his wife to stop seeing the psychiatrist failed, he became panicky.

It was apparent that living with an emotionally disturbed wife for several years was not a problem for this man. The hazardous situation that threatened him was the possibility that she would get well. When this obvious fact became clear to him in the first interview, he decided not to return for a second visit.

However, the more his wife improved, the more upset and tense he became. He made an effort to see his wife's psychiatrist in order to convince him to stop seeing her but he was unsuccessful. He felt angry and returned to the agency for help, but by then he had stopped working and appeared to be depressed. He described himself as being discouraged, unable to sleep, and feeling tired and guilty.

The point is that this man developed anxiety and became angry at the time when he faced a hazardous environmental situation. Unable to deal with it, he grew more anxious. At this point he reached a state of emotional crisis. When he was unable to convince his wife to stop seeing her psychiatrist he became panicky. The failure to continue to visit the agency contributed to his difficulties. His inability to cope with the crisis aggravated his condition. By the time he returned to the agency psychiatric symptoms were in evidence. He was now depressed.

His attempt to deal with his crisis by running away did not help, nor did the turning of his anger inward. These were maladaptive reactions to the situation and were responsible for the symptom of depression. By staying home, and not working, he isolated himself from the outside world, and was temporarily incapacitated. This regressive behavior helped him mobilize all his resources. He soon returned to the agency. There he was helped to reexamine and eventually to overcome his difficulties. Only then was he able to return to a state of emotional equilibrium.

Hazardous situations are usually stressful. Maladaptive psychological reactions to them can, at times, lead to painful feelings. Following some precipitating event, these feelings are suddenly intensified and in turn lead to the development of an emotional crisis, which emerges before the clear-cut appearance of the psychiatric symptoms. At such a time an individual struggles with all his available resources to overcome his distress. His ultimate success or failure are crucial for his mental health.

In observing individuals who are facing emotional crises, we distinguish between the painful state and the reaction to the painful state. The motives for the reaction are invariably the same: the repetitive attempt to alleviate the painful state. On the other hand, the means used to achieve this objective differ from one individual to another.

Several terms have been used which require definition: a stressful situation is one which elicits painful emotions in an individual, and a hazardous situation is a difficult or dangerous situation that becomes stressful to some individuals and not to others. One can present a long list of such universally dangerous situations. The threat of nuclear annihilation, water and air pollution, and continued increase in the world population may be too general. More specifically, the Cuban or Berlin Crises, the Vietnam or Middle East wars have recently been in our minds. In the past, World War II, the 1918-1919 influenza pandemic, the Black Death — all these threatened large sections of society with extinction. During such times it is understandable if we become upset and anxious and desire that something be done immediately to relieve this dreadful state of affairs.

Some individuals may see spies round any corner or may decide to take matters into their own hands and kill a leader whom they view as the cause of all this difficulty. Others may be so paralyzed with fear that they become temporarily incapacitated and may be unable to function. They are casualties of these hazardous situations which have become too stressful for them to endure.

Hazardous situations may also arise from within the individual. Adolescence, for example, is not stressful to everybody, yet some young people develop emotional difficulties during adolescence which may lead to quick deterioration and the onset of psychiatric symptoms. Several years ago I saw, at a mental health agency in an upper middle class suburb of Boston, 108 individuals who were in a state of emotional crisis. Of these, 84 were women and 24 men — a ratio approximately 4 to 1. Ninety-five were married, 13 were not (10 were single, 2 divorced, 1 widowed). Most of them were young. For example, 70 percent ranged in age from 20 to 50 years and 20 percent were in their teens. Of the remaining 6, 4 were in their fifties and the other two were 61 and 67, respectively. Protestants outnumbered Catholics by 3 to 1. Twenty-five belonged to family units in which at least two other members were interviewed. They were referred by friends, family doctors, schoolteachers, clergymen, and the local hospital and family agency. Fifty-two were self-referred.

The hazardous situations which gave rise to anxiety and led to an emotional crisis included: loss of a member of the family by separation, illness, or death; disturbed behavior (excessively passive or aggressive) of a member of the family, usually a child; physical or mental illness of another member of their immediate circle; a new arrival in the family orbit such as a new baby or a sibling returned from service with the armed forces; a change in civil status such as marriage, a move into a new community, and a change of roles forced upon an individual by changes which affected another member of the family. Other situations involved a new job, retirement, or unemployment; entrance into college or professional school; and isolation of the family from the community or entrance of their child into kindergarten or school. All these were environmental situations which motivated those individuals to seek help. Hazards arising from within the individual himself were physical illness, incapacitating injury, puberty, adolescence, pregnancy, climacterium, and old age.

A painful state is an unpleasant emotional state in which anxiety, sorrow, anger, and fear predominate and which usually arises as a result of stressful or hazardous situations. A reaction is a response to a stimulus that arises from within the individual. Reaction is used here in a somewhat broader sense than the term "psychological defense mechanism." A successful or adaptive reaction is one which, at times of hazardous situations or emotional crises, does not give rise to painful states. An unsuccessful or maladaptive reaction is an inadequate reaction which, at times of hazardous situations, *does* give rise to painful states which continue to predominate. A chief complaint is the reason chosen by the individual for seeking professional help. It may or may not reflect the true hazardous situation faced by him at that time. It may be, for example, some sort of justification for his visit to a mental health agency, a clinic, or a doctor's private office. Some of the 108 individuals said they had come only to please the referring physician or teacher. "The school principal says my daughter should get better grades"; "My nephew is insane; would it help if he visited your agency?"; "My son cries and is unwilling to go to school"; "My husband cannot get along with my younger boy"; "My clergyman thinks I should consult you about my daughter's rebellious behavior." It was obvious, however, that they had problems of their own which it was the task of the interviewer to assess.

Although the individual's fear and nervousness were apparent, they at first minimized anxiety about some of their complaints but soon admitted that such feelings existed and that the attempts to deal with them had been unsuccessful. Some visitors to the agency, on the other hand, admitted right away being anxious and disturbed about the behavior of another member of their family: "I am upset about my four-year-old boy's thumb sucking"; "I fear that my son is on the verge of running away from home. What shall I do?" Others openly worried about themselves: "I feel that the top of my head is going to fly off"; "I wonder why my hands always shake when I go out on a date"; "I feel at times that life is not worth while"; "I am worried about the failures of my three previous marriages. I am getting married for the fourth time in another week."

A precipitating factor is usually an environmental event that brings about a change in painful feelings. It is usually apparent that within the recent past the precipitating factor acted in a way to bring the anxiety from a somewhat dormant state into the open. Thus, it may initiate an emotional crisis, it may signal the beginning of a psychotic break, or it may act as a final crowning blow which may lead to a suicide attempt. Most often, however, it motivates the individual to seek help. A talk with a family doctor, for example, acted as a pre-cipitating factor for some individuals and motivated them to seek psychiatric help. Interviews with teachers, visits to clergymen, lawyers, nurses, job supervisors, or even a talk with a policeman or a friend may be the precipitating factor. Sometimes the interview at a mental health agency may act as a precipitating factor for getting another member of the family to visit the agency. A visit to a private psychiatrist or social worker, impending examinations at school, physical examinations, quarrels with a relative, new jobs, admissions or discharges from a hospital, meetings of League of Women Voters or P.T.A.'s or Cub Scouts, engagements, journeys, possibility of a child's expulsion from school — all these situations acted as precipitating factors which intensified the anxiety. But it is anxiety — this raw material which acts as a signal to alert us to future dangers — that is responsible for our psychological defense mechanisms which protect us from the vicissitudes of everyday life. This seemed to be the main motivating force for most of these individuals, and it was with the hope of relief from excessive anxiety that they came to the mental health agency.

The defense mechanisms used in an attempt to handle anxiety varied according to the personalities of the individuals. The need to call on additional defense mechanisms became apparent when the anxiety could not be properly handled and the awareness of the painful emotions became intensified. At such a time they were in a state of emotional crisis.

An analogy may illustrate what I mean: In chemical quantitative analysis there is a point when one drop of base, added to a colorless solution which contains phenolphthalein turns the whole fluid suddenly into a bright red color. The last drop of base is the precipitating factor; the red solution is the emotional crisis for all to see.

As a turning point for better or for worse, the emotional crisis may stimulate the individual to utilize a new set of reactions in an attempt to overcome it successfully and return to a previously existing state of emotional equilibrium. The crisis may not be dealt with adequately, however. In fact, it may further intensify the pain and, by use of maladaptive compromises, give rise to the production of psychiatric symptoms which, if they become fixed, may eventually take the form of a full-blown neurosis. Thus, an emotional crisis is a powerful internalized stimulus demanding further reactions. There are several factors involved in assessing its intensity which will be discussed later.

Some individuals cling to, and depend exclusively on, the

environment to solve their crises. They tend to take action haphazardly, hoping that in this way they can get relief. "I must act," they say. "I must make non-negotiable demands" they cry. So familiar and fashionable nowadays! As a result they may attempt to manipulate the environment, they may take precipitous action with disastrous results to themselves and others, or they may retreat to the inflexible protection of their house, and they may rely on their financial resources exclusively to weather an emotional storm. All these maneuvers may be successful for the time being, but these individuals still remain vulnerable. If they find themselves in a different environment, however, where they cannot use action nor depend upon those materialistic resources, they will invariably start to crumble. Thus, depending upon something outside of one's control, which is not "built in" in one's own individual character, is always dangerous. Of course there are those who use different, but exclusively pathological, reactions. Paranoid patients, for example, blame others for their own deficiencies, thus absolving themselves from any inadequacy or guilt. Some suicidal individuals manipulate the environment dramatically in order to go on living (see Case 2 in Chapter 2). All these are usually unsuccessful ways of coping with emotional crises. Finally, it should be emphasized that an emotional crisis in one individual may create a hazardous situation for other members of his family or his immediate circle of friends.

Out of the variety of emotional problems presented by these 108 individuals, I have chosen the following cases to illustrate the hazardous situations, the anxieties, the precipitating factors, the emotional crises, and finally the reactions which were used to cope with them.

CASE 2. A twenty-three-year-old law student developed tuberculosis, which forced him to give up law school for a period of two years. After his discharge from the hospital his mother was overprotective. She constantly warned him not to catch cold, not to sit in a draft, and she wanted him to get more sleep. When he decided to take a trip to Europe before returning to school she objected. He became upset by all these solicitations, actively reduplicated his preparations to leave, and considered marrying his current girl friend. When his mother failed in her attempts to persuade him to change his mind about Europe, she tried to plan the whole trip for him. He reacted to this by being bewildered at first, then becoming anxious, and finally angry. Two years of being dependent and lying in bed had been enough for him; he now wanted to be on his own. He talked to a family friend who suggested a consultation with a psychiatrist.

The night before coming for his first visit he quarreled with his mother when he announced to her his plans to be married. She burst into tears and stated emphatically that she was not going to allow any woman to take her son away from her "after two years of separation." It was this statement that made him furious and prompted the thought of packing and leaving right then. He soon changed his mind, however. He decided to come to the mental health agency for help the following day.

Talking about his difficulties with his mother, he could quickly discover that his independent overactivity was a reaction to her overprotectiveness. Yet he also realized that he enjoyed her care of him and recognized his wish to depend upon her. He decided to talk things over with her once more. When he returned the following week, he said that a compromise had been reached. He had decided to postpone his marriage for a while and continued his plans to spend a month in a small town in Spain, which he had always wanted to do, and another month visiting various countries and following his mother's itinerary. He said that he understood better his mother's worries about him after such a long separation and felt sure that he loved her. He asserted that there was no need on his part to deny with such vehemence his long-standing dependence on his mother. A modus vivendi had been found.

The whole situation is quite simple in this case. A well-integrated young man threatened by the hazard of enforced passivity and faced with his dependent wishes, develops an emotional crisis as a result of his mother's overprotective attitude. He considers flight as a way out. A talk with a friend precipitates his visit to a mental health agency, where during the interview he develops a more objective view of his difficulties. He reacts by reaching a satisfactory compromise between his conflicting wishes to be both dependent and independent. In this way he is able to maintain both his relationship with his mother and his self-esteem intact.

CASE 3. A middle-aged nurse, mother of two daughters, came to the mental health agency complaining of being "at the end of her rope." She said that throughout the many years of marriage her husband had been fearful of people, locked the doors in every room of their house, always looked under the beds at night, was convinced at times that everyone was against him, and was always in a perpetual state of turmoil. She also went into a detailed description of her husband's toilet habits. He always kept stools in three different toilets, which he flushed periodically, one at a time. She and the daughters had to share the fourth bathroom. Ten years previously her husband had had a "nervous break-down," at which time he became withdrawn and had stopped working. During that period she took good care of him all by herself, and he soon recovered.

Throughout all the years of what might be thought of as a stressful marriage, she had lived happily by denying the seriousness of her husband's queer habits and by saying to herself, "All people have peculiarities." Her husband was successful financially. He used his house as an office. He invested wisely and amassed a large fortune. His wife was able to point to his financial wisdom and rationalized his queer habits by considering him "a genius." She seemed to be unaware of the extremes in his behavior.

On the occasion of their daughter's graduation from high school she decided that the whole family should celebrate and take a cruise to the Caribbean. Her husband was very reluctant to agree at first, but after much pressure from her he finally capitulated. Complications developed as soon as they embarked, which might have been expected, when her husband realized that he had to share the toilet with other people in the next cabin. She had made elaborate arrangements to anticipate this situation, but it appeared that there were too many passengers on the ship, so that they were forced to accept this particular cabin. Her husband immediately became suspicious. He started to behave in a very peculiar way and attracted the attention of the neighbors by his insistence that they should not flush the toilet. On one occasion he was the object of much laughter and ridicule when, fearing that his clothes had become contaminated, he ran nude from the ship's swimming pool to his cabin. At that particular time, when his wife overheard the passengers speaking about "that crazy man," she became alarmed. Later on, after one of the daughters had had an argument with her father, she turned to her mother and said, "I cannot see how you could have lived with such a madman for twenty years." At this point she became very upset and started to visualize the realities of the situation.

What seems to have given rise to the anxiety in this woman was the sudden realization that her husband was really sick. She immediately took steps to arrange for the whole family to return home as soon as possible. The thought that her husband might be mentally ill lingered, and her anxiety persisted. She decided to nurse her husband, as she had done ten years previously, but this time he reacted in a very different way. He angrily accused her of purposely arranging the trip in such a manner as to expose him to a hostile world and of plotting to put him at the mercy of evil people who were against him. It seemed that, for the first time in their marriage, he turned his rage against her, and on one occasion, he actually grabbed her by the neck and tried to choke her. It was at this point that she became panicky and turned to her minister for help. This visit precipitated her coming to the mental health agency. "If I could only stop thinking about my husband being angry at me, everything would be all right." She exclaimed, "I have tried to, but I cannot, and I am thinking of divorce for the first time in my married life."

In this case, as long as this woman's husband expressed anger against others, she was not threatened; but as a result of the hazardous trip she developed anxiety, which increased when the husband's hostility was turned against her. She was in a state of emotional crisis, unable to tolerate it, unable to deal with it in her old familiar way of denying or rationalizing it, hence she started to think of taking action in the form of divorce as a solution to her problem.

CASE 4. A thirty-five-year-old married schoolteacher, mother of an eight-year-old boy, came to the agency complaining of anxiety associated with the visit of her mother-in-law. She was an intelligent, pleasant woman, a college graduate, who related well to the interviewer. She described her marriage as being a happy one up to the time when her mother-in-law decided to come from England and visit them. Since this was the first encounter with her husband's mother, she made every effort to get along well with her; but when the visitor announced her plans for an indefinite stay, she became apprehensive. Her tension increased when she was criticized for teaching school rather than staying at home "as every good mother should." When the mother-in-law started to discipline the patient's son and commented that it was fortunate that the boy had his grandmother to take care of him, she became very angry. Her efforts to discuss the whole situation with her old-fashioned visitor were met with no success. At this point, she started to feel inadequate. She developed nightmares. Her work at school suffered, and she could not concentrate; but what upset her most was that she began to be afraid to walk alone in the streets, particularly at night. She appealed to her husband for help, but he was hesitant about annoying his mother. It was a quarrel with her husband over his refusal to ask his mother, point blank, to leave that made her decide to visit the agency and to stop teaching school.

Her husband also was interviewed, and an attempt was made to explain to him his wife's predicament. He seemed to be willing to cooperate. His wife was seen on four occasions over a period of eight months. On the second visit, she announced that her husband had been unsuccessful in convincing his mother to go.

Her husband was seen again. Although he had not been able to confront his mother, he was angry at her because she had started an affair with a man of her own age. He was appalled by this, particularly when his mother insinuated that she was seriously considering divorce in order to marry this man.

It was the patient who became determined, however, to ask her mother-in-law to leave. She felt she was in better control of the situation and was furthermore encouraged because this woman was spending less time complaining about the patient's inadequacies and more time with her lover. The confrontation between these two ladies was timed perfectly. It occurred when signs had appeared that the mother-in-law's affair was not going along so well. At this point the patient suggested to her visitor that it was time she returned to England. To her surprise there was no opposition. When she was interviewed six months later, all was well. She was symptom free and had returned to her teaching position. She, as well as her husband and her son, were happy.

It was clear that this woman, who had functioned so well in the past, was unable to cope with her emotional crisis. In her own way, however, this very failure helped her to overcome her difficulties by allowing her to concentrate all her resources on the solution of her emotional problem. The phobias isolated her from the outside world, kept her at home, and helped her to disregard the accusations that she had been a bad housekeeper and a part-time mother. Giving up her job reinforced temporarily her assumption of the central role in her household and keeping control of her son. Successful utilization of her environmental resources, such as the mental health agency and the support of her husband, also helped. She was encouraged to take matters into her own hands and to solve her difficulties.

The unsuccessful attempts of all these individuals to face hazardous situations led to the development of emotional crises because of the use of maladaptive psychological reactions. It was only when they were able to deal with and overcome these crises that they were able to function again. Keeping my definitions of the terms used and the case material in mind, I would like to conceptualize the process which leads to an emotional crisis in the following model.

At first an individual is in an unpainful state, but, exposed to stress arising from either within or without, he enters a painful state. A successful reaction to the stressful situation will eliminate anxiety, thus eradicating the painful state, while an unsuccessful reaction will intensify it. It is possible, however, that an individual may temporarily reach a precarious balance and remain in a painful state. The individual who fails to return to an unpainful state because of his inability to utilize environmental resources successfully or to mobilize adequate individual reactions remains vulnerable. A threatening outside event acts as a precipitating factor and gives rise to an intensification, or a change for the worse, of the already painful condition. It is at this point that the individual enters a state of emotional crisis, which has already been defined. Here again there are two possible reactions to the crisis: successful, by eliminating it, and unsuccessful, by further aggravating and intensifying it. The emotional crisis thus has become a powerful internalized stimulus, demanding alleviation or satisfactory adjustment for the better or leading to further deterioration for the worse. The question must be raised, then, as to what happens if the emotional crisis is not resolved. The patient may develop temporary psychiatric symptoms which could eventually crystallize into a neurosis. But a neurosis is a halfway measure! It is a solution of sorts but, indeed, it is a vulnerable state which may at any time be altered for the worse.

Here, for example, is what happens with some suicidal individuals. Unable to deal with their emotional crises, their painful states become intensified and at such a time the idea of suicide may occur to them as a way out. They now exist in a state of precarious adjustment. The pressures continue, however. They interfere with the usefulness of the patient's defense mechanisms and slowly push them to an even more painful state with a change in the intensity of their emotions. As a reaction to this, they make a few futile attempts but they are unable to deal with the situation which gives rise to acutely painful emotions or an acutely painful state. A precipitating event may further change the form of emotions or symptoms, and they now seriously consider suicide. This state can be called "autoktonism" (from the Greek *autokteno*, meaning self-killing), which is a state of mind in individuals who are about to commit suicide as recognized by trained observers.[1] The denouement is reached when the patient finally uses the one and only possible reaction that seems available to him — suicide.

Extreme as this example may be, it shows the steps taken by individuals who are ultimately unable to deal with their emotional crises. They must decide whether they should use all their resources to cope with this crisis, even if it should temporarily incapacitate them and would be at the expense of their general, overall functioning, or they should attempt to deal with both situations at the same time. Note that in Cases 1 and 4 the efforts to do both failed. The crises deepened, and symptoms started to appear. It was when the individuals involved concentrated all their resources to overcome the emotional crisis that they succeeded. It was only then that they could resume their everyday activities.

An individual's ability to use flexibly all sorts of reactions, even pathological ones, and his concentration on resolving the emotional crisis may be a useful asset in his efforts to return to an unpainful state. On the other hand, an attempt to cope rigidly with the demands and hazards of everyday life and to use inflexible reactions to deal with emotional crises leads invariably to progressive failure and ensuing disaster. The young adolescent who is depressed one day, anxious the next, running away on the third, and dependent on the fourth is better off than the adolescent who rigidly clings to only one way of dealing with his stress.

The role of emotional crisis has been described for programs of preventive intervention. H. C. Schulberg and Shelton[2] emphasize that a probability formulation of crisis depends upon the occurrence of a hazardous event and that an individual will be exposed and will be vulnerable to it. They review a variety of anticipatory and participatory intervention techniques and suggest guidelines for their selection in averting a crisis. In my opinion, in the final analysis, an emotional crisis is an ever-changing idiosyncratic experience and, as such, is potentially valuable or potentially dangerous, but is invariably fascinating. It offers an opportunity to reverse the maladaptive processes and to restore a badly deranged emotional equilibrium.

The description of normal people is difficult. There are no diagnoses that one can use — no tags, no labels. The usual nosological criteria are of little help. This concept of emotional crisis is a dynamic one. It gives us furthermore a fleeting glimpse of both healthy and emotionally unhealthy human beings and a chance to describe their psychodynamic continuum. The ways in which they face, struggle against, and overcome emotional crises is interesting to observe; the ways by which we can help them in their efforts are significant in their implications, and will be discussed in the following chapters.

4

TWO DIFFERENT KINDS OF PSYCHOTHERAPY OF SHORT DURATION

Therapeutic techniques aimed at shortening the length of psychotherapy without interfering with its efficacy offer advantages which obviously require no comment. In this chapter I shall present a conceptual frame of reference for two kinds of psychotherapy of short duration[1] which may be appropriate for the needs of two entirely different groups of patients. Who are, then, the individuals who can benefit from these two kinds of short-term psychotherapy which can be considered the treatment of choice for their specific emotional difficulties?

At this point one may be tempted to exaggerate in order to simplify the discussion and divide psychiatric patients into two large categories: those who, because of genetic, bio-chemical, developmental, or environmental factors, or a combination of all of them, have been unable to develop adequately and have attained only a precarious level of emotional functioning. Because of these predispositions, these patients have poor interpersonal relations, are barely able to deal with the vicissitudes of everyday life, and have lifelong emotional difficulties. At times of stress, they decompensate rapidly and require immediate assistance.

In contrast to this group, there are those individuals who have developed adequate strengths of character and are able to deal with the realities of the world, which enables them to function fairly well. At times of stress, they also may become temporarily incapacitated, but the kinds of emotional problems which they develop are well circumscribed, and their complaints are specific and clear cut and do not interfere radically with their overall functioning.

Because they are offered to these different groups of patients and are technically dissimilar, psychotherapies of short duration may be divided into two types: anxiety-suppressive, or supportive, and anxiety-provoking, or dynamic.

Anxiety-Suppressive, or Supportive Psychotherapy

The aim of anxiety-suppressive, or supportive psychotherapy is to decrease or eliminate anxiety by use of supportive therapeutic techniques, such as reassurance, environmental manipulation, hospitalization, or appropriate medication. This type of treatment may be prolonged, but for all intents and purposes a selected group of patients suffering from severe psychiatric disorders, such as some types of severe character disorders or certain kinds of frankly psychotic illnesses, may benefit from "brief anxiety-suppressive psychotherapy," lasting anywhere from two months to one year. It is also possible to use similar therapeutic interventions to help some of these patients during an acutely critical time with only a few interviews timed appropriately over one or two months. Such an approach is referred to as "crisis support." Long-term anxiety suppressive psychotherapy is commonly used to help seriously disturbed patients.

These time intervals should not be considered arbitrary but are mentioned here simply as guidelines.

Brief "Anxiety-Suppressive" Psychotherapy

Patients with lifelong emotional difficulties may be offered this kind of psychotherapy if they are selected according to the following criteria: (1) ability to maintain a job, (2) a strong appeal for help to overcome their emotional difficulties, (3) recognition that the symptoms are psychological in origin, and (4) willingness to cooperate with psychotherapy. Every effort should be made to evaluate such patients quickly and on an individual basis, trying to assess how precarious is the underlying character structure, how serious is the emotional illness, and how the patient who is suffering from it is able to function, despite its presence.

Requirements and Technique

The requirements for this kind of brief psychotherapy involve seeing the patient in face-to-face interviews once, twice, or several times a week, lasting anywhere from a few minutes to more than an hour if it is necessary. A flexible approach regarding interviews depends upon the patient's needs, as far as the therapeutic technique is concerned.

The therapist makes an attempt to establish rapport with the patient as soon as possible and allows him to tell his story freely without interruptions. If this tends to make him anxious, however, the therapist tries to reassure him by changing the subject or by choosing to question the patient about his past, social, or medical history. He tries to convince the patient throughout this time that he is eager to help and reassures him that everything will be done to provide him with symptomatic relief.

He uses appropriate medication whenever it is indicated, and he makes an effort to alter and decrease the pressures on the patient arising in his environment by utilizing the aid of social agencies or by seeking assistance from the members of the patient's family. He "lends himself" to the patient if necessary, by taking over some of his decision-making functions for a short while during this crucial time and by offering recommendations for the patient to follow. He encourages the patient at other times to take specific action under certain circumstances and gives him concrete and detailed advice on how to go about achieving what he desires. He helps the patient to review and understand the ways to deal with his feelings when faced with hazardous situations which gave rise to his emotional crisis and may be responsible for his decompensation. He predicts the patient's future behavior on the basis of his past performance and, in this way, prepares him to

rehearse his reactions in order to avoid future difficulties.
Here is an example which illustrates some of these points:

A twenty-four-year-old man who had been an overt homosexual since the age of sixteen entered the psychiatry clinic complaining of panic, inability to work, and thoughts of killing himself as a way out of his misery. These symptoms appeared immediately after his homosexual partner, with whom he had been living, left him after an argument. He gave a history of lifelong emotional difficulties. He had been admitted to mental hospitals on two occasions because of suicidal attempts. Both his parents had died in an automobile accident when he was two years old, and he was brought up by relatives. He was an intelligent high school graduate who had fairly steady work patterns and seemed to be eager for help.

In twice-a-week brief anxiety-suppressive psychotherapy an attempt was made to relieve the acute distress over the loss of his boy friend. He was complimented for seeking help in the clinic rather than resorting to suicide. His reaction patterns to previous losses were reviewed. The prospect of future losses was discussed in detail, and he was helped to prepare himself to deal with them. He was able to talk about his angry feelings for having been abandoned. After a while he felt better, returned to work, and soon established a new homosexual relationship. In four months he was symptom free.

Follow-up

We have not studied the follow-up findings of this type of psychotherapy extensively, but our current observations point to (1) marked symptomatic relief; (2) some ability to avoid the situations which gave rise to the symptoms which brought the patient to the clinic; (3) an attitude of viewing the clinic, rather than the therapist, as the supportive agent; (4) no evidence of psychodynamic change; and (5) a tendency to return to the hospital at times of future difficulties.

Crisis Support

Crisis support therapy, which is also offered to seriously disturbed patients, lasts up to about two months. It attempts to eliminate as quickly as possible the factors responsible for the patient's crisis which led to his decompensation, and it helps him overcome the acutely traumatic situation in which he finds himself. Successful utilization of environmental resources, such as agencies and hospital clinics, or specific individuals — such as family doctors, ministers, teachers, educators, friends, and relatives — can be invaluable in helping these patients to overcome their difficulties. In some sense, also, these individuals are in strategic positions because they usually see the patient before the psychiatrist sees him and are able by their proximity with him to steer him accurately to the place where he can get help.

The emphasis then should be on using anxiety-suppressive techniques. The patient may be seen frequently for short intervals, or he may be hospitalized. Drugs should be given freely. The follow-up findings are similar to those obtained in "brief anxiety-suppressive psychotherapy."

Case Material

Here is a double example of crisis support therapy.

A husband and wife came to the mental health agency together. The wife was seen by the psychiatrist and the husband by a social worker. On their way to the agency they had a quarrel. The wife, blushing and trembling, talked rapidly and, at times, almost incoherently. She told of being fearful of her husband and of being suspicious of men in general. She mentioned a plot against her life. She was twenty-nine years old and an only child. Her mother had died when she was six months old. Her father was still living, but she was not close to him. She married when she was an adolescent and, after the birth of her first child, she became nervous and was unable to cope with the responsibilities of bringing up her child. Trying hard and almost desperate as a result of her young son's demands, she became more and more meticulous in her housework and started to do compulsive acts, such as washing the sink or the bathtub repetitively. "I gave the appearance of being a perfect housewife, yet I could see things slipping in my household," she said. She had three more children, and during her fifth pregnancy she felt "at the end of the rope." "Cracks started to show in my establishment but I still tried to keep up a front; but soon I started to have fears about being sick and about dying. I thought of suicide, but I still tried to keep up pretenses."

After the delivery of her fifth child she developed an infection. When she returned home she was exhausted and was unable to breast feed this baby, as she had done with all her other children. It was at this point that she became suspicious of everyone and of men in particular. She claimed to have come to the agency just to complain about her husband.

Her husband, in turn, talked about his wife's "mental illness" and was eager to give his side of the marital conflict. He said that his wife was an excellent housekeeper, but she had become upset when she was unable to take care of the children, particularly during the last few months. He was very upset by her condition.

The wife returned to the agency the next day. She was very agitated. She refused to go to a mental hospital and emphasized that only her minister or her father-in-law — the only two people she trusted — could persuade her to be admitted. Arrangements were made to have these two people present during her third visit. Together they were able to convince her that she needed help and that the local mental hospital was the most suitable place for her.

She was treated in a mental hospital for a few months. After her discharge she was seen supportively by her own doctor at the hospital for a while. Soon after, she was able to resume her household duties.

Her husband was seen supportively a few times. Despite his long history of emotional difficulties, he was able to care for his children alone. He was visited at his home by the social worker and was seen in the process of running his household. It was interesting to watch the older children "in action" taking care of the younger ones, although they ranged in age from eight years to four months. He did a competent job, and the children appeared happy. It was easy to motivate him to seek further psychiatric help for his own emotional difficulties.

The agency kept in contact with the family for two years. The wife, despite her serious difficulties, seemed to be able again to deal with the situation, and both husband and wife were doing quite well.

In viewing this case in retrospect one may observe that the wife's attempts to face the hazards of repeated pregnancies had failed. Her rigid obsessive compulsive efforts to keep up pretenses slowly disintegrated, and her inability to adjust to the pressures of the outside world progressively led to a deterioration which finally required hospitalization.

The husband, also, was in a critical state, but his ability to take over his wife's duties at home and to work with a psychiatrist in crisis support helped him from regressing, and enabled him to keep the family together until his wife's return.

Long-Term Anxiety-Suppressive Psychotherapy

As mentioned before, anxiety-suppressive psychotherapy can be long term. In my book *Ascent from Chaos*[2] I have described the development of an anaclitic relationship which was life-saving to a seriously disturbed patient with psychosomatic difficulties, who was alcoholic, addicted to narcotics, and who also made repeated suicidal attempts and tried to choke another patient. In a sense, allowing a patient to rely completely on his therapist, which is the nature of the anaclitic relationship, and having all his dependent needs and exaggerated demands satisfied can be viewed as an extremely unusual form of long-term anxiety-supportive psychotherapy.

Predicting future behavior on the basis of past performance and teaching the patient to rehearse his reactions to anxiety-producing situations has been described as a technical point of brief anxiety-suppressive psychotherapy. In a modified way it is also utilized in anxiety-provoking psychotherapy and will be discussed later on.

It can also be used in long-term anxiety-suppressive psychotherapy to help certain seriously disturbed chronic paranoid patients. The case histories of three such patients will be presented, and some of the theoretical and technical aspects of these cases will be discussed briefly.

All three patients had certain similar features. They were middle-aged married women, with young dependent daughters. They were fond of their husbands at one time, but after they had been threatened repeatedly with separation, they developed paranoid ideas which soon turned into delusions. They maintained good relations with their children, however, despite their psychotic symptoms and clung to them desperately without involving them in their paranoid systems. After their husbands abandoned them, two of these patients appeared in court and obtained both a divorce and full custody of their daughters. Although they complained to their children constantly about men in general and their husbands in particular and related their sexual experiences, the children did not seem to pay much attention to these confessions and there was no evidence that they were adversely influenced by them. The way in which these women interacted with their therapists was reminiscent of the way they related to their children.

CONCEPTUAL FRAME OF REFERENCE

Case Material

The following three cases demonstrate a specialized kind of long-term anxiety-suppressive psychotherapy.

CASE 1. A thirty-five-year-old mother of five was brought to the psychiatry clinic by a neighbor because she was confused, tense, and expressed paranoid delusions. Five days previously, she had discovered that her husband had had several extramarital affairs and she quarreled with him. When he asked her for a separation, she became furious and threatened to kill him. Frightened, he packed during the night and departed. Upon discovering his disappearance the next day, she became confused and started to fear that her house was being watched, that the food was poisoned, and that her husband would return to take the children away from her.

During the interview she was restless, tense, and fearful and expressed paranoid delusions about her husband, but after a while, she was able to give a fairly coherent history. When she was seen for a second interview she had calmed down considerably. She was assigned to a psychiatrist for long-term anxiety-suppressive psychotherapy in the hope of avoiding hospitalization. Paranoid ideas predominated at first, but after she was actively reassured that her children would not be taken away, she felt better. She improved so much in a few months that she was able to take night courses, obtain a job, and support her family.

The therapist concentrated on trying to teach her to anticipate situations which were likely to produce confusion, and anxiety, and to give rise to paranoid thinking. When he asked her to describe what might happen during her husband's periodic visits, she was totally unable to anticipate such a situation. It was the therapist's task to describe, on the basis of previous information, what might transpire. He would go on as follows, "Last time, as soon as your husband arrived, you thought that he brought the police with him to take your children away. You told me that you got mad and wanted to kill him. I suspect that the same thing will happen next time he visits you. You may also start thinking that he poisoned the food and that he turned the neighbors against you. The thought may even cross your mind that I am deceiving you. Now, you must prepare yourself for all this to happen." When, in the next interview, the patient exclaimed, "Doctor, are you reading my mind? It happened the way you said it would. How did you know? Was it magic?" He simply answered that he had predicted her behavior on the basis of information she had given to him in previous interviews. Teaching the patient to anticipate such a situation had to be repeated over and over, and the doctor had to dispel the notion of magic.

After three years the patient felt secure enough to undertake a move to another state, where her relatives had offered her a free house. She managed her children very well and seemed satisfied with her life. She also corresponded frequently with her therapist and her social worker. In her letters she described in detail her elaborate preparations to anticipate and to avoid trouble.

CASE 2. A fifty-year-old woman had been hospitalized on two occasions with the diagnosis of "paranoid psychosis." She had three illegitimate children who were given away for adoption, and she was considered to be "a problem" in the community in which she lived. A man who married her, soon deserted her, and she was living with her daughter, of whom he was the father. She was in constant fear, however, that he would return to take his daughter away from her, because everyone considered her to be an unfit mother.

When she came to the clinic she was confused, tense, and expressed paranoid delusions. The resident who interviewed her wanted to hospitalize her, but he changed his mind when she pleaded with him not to do so, for fear that she might lose custody of her daughter. An appointment was made for the following day, by which time she had felt somewhat better. She received anxiety-suppressive psychotherapy for the next two years, and she managed fairly well. When her therapist was drafted into the army, she decompensated and became acutely paranoid, having been unable to anticipate the separation. She also developed a peptic ulcer. She recovered quickly, however, and was willing to trust the new psychiatrist who was assigned to her. He helped her learn to anticipate separations, including his own, and in contrast, there was only a slight increase in her paranoid ideation after he left.

She used the interviews with the third therapist to talk about her sexual experiences, which she called "sadistic orgies," and at the end she felt invariably better. On one occasion she brought her eleven-year-old daughter to the clinic to introduce her to the therapist. During the interview, when she started as usual to describe her "orgies," the little girl interrupted her mother angrily, "Mummy, stop it," she said, "Don't talk like that in front of the doctor." The patient promptly apologized, and smiling, she added, "You see, Doctor, Mary has much better sense than I do." It appeared that the child was aware of her mother's mental illness and had learned to live with it. She loved her mother despite her faults, but she had also learned to protect her. Getting used to her mother's tirades was the price she had to pay for keeping their relationship intact.

The patient was followed for a long time and was seen on an infrequent basis. She also managed to obtain a divorce and full custody of her daughter. After an absence of several years from the Boston area she returned to the clinic to announce that her daughter, now twenty-one years old, was going to be married. She said that she had anticipated their separation and added significantly, "Aren't these the times of difficulty when I should return to the clinic?"

CASE 3. A forty-six-year-old married mother of a ten-year-old girl came to the clinic in a state of acute decompensation. She complained that people were laughing at her, making indecent advances to her. She also claimed that she heard her husband's voice accusing her of sexual promiscuity. The onset of her present illness had followed the death of an elderly woman with whom she had been very close, and the announcement that her husband had accepted an assignment with the army overseas. She became upset and pleaded with him to reconsider, but when he refused she felt panicky and confused. Soon after his departure she deteriorated rapidly and developed auditory hallucinations.

The patient was an obese, deaf, unkempt woman, with psoriatic lesions, looking older than her stated age. She was tense and expressed her anger about her husband. She was put on Trifluoperazine hydrochloride and was assigned to a social worker and a psychiatrist.

Six months after the start of her psychotherapy she found out that her husband was in an army hospital dying of cancer. She was encouraged to talk about her feelings and expectations and to make preparations for his death. This she was able to do, and when he died, she regressed somewhat, was able to grieve, but she did not deteriorate appreciably. In her interviews she talked warmly about her relationship with her daughter. In a letter to her psychiatrist, she stated, "I taught my daughter to be a good girl early. No one taught me anything. I was green about men and sex. The other day when I told her that the television man made a sexual pass at me she said, "Come on, Mummy, don't exaggerate." I laughed and laughed. She has a better sense of humor than I do. "You're right, honey," I said, "I did exaggerate, but I tried to teach you just as the doctor does with me."

After her daughter won a scholarship to college, she developed a few paranoid ideas, which soon subsided. With a telephone, which was installed with the help of the hospital's social service department, mother and daughter were able to keep in touch with each other. Four years later, after her daughter graduated from college and announced to the patient that she was going to Europe to be married, she decompensated temporarily and had to be hospitalized for awhile. At present she is living alone.

Discussion

It appears that all three patients, unable to anticipate separation, became acutely anxious, angry, and confused. These feelings intensified the patients' difficulties. In this critical state, by using exclusively such defense mechanisms as denial, distortion, and particularly projection, they developed paranoid symptoms. On the verge of collapse, they were in danger of losing their dependent children. For all concerned, the mental health hazards of such a situation cannot be overemphasized.

Since projection plays the major role in paranoid symptom formation, a distinction should be made between two kinds of projection — primary and secondary. In primary projection, the patient is totally unaware of what he is doing, while in secondary projection he is partly aware. An analogy may serve to illustrate this point. A child playing with a rubber ball with an elastic attached to it may throw the ball and the elastic at someone else, thus losing control of it, or he may throw the ball and hold the elastic, thus keeping partial control of the ball. The former happens in primary projection, and the latter in secondary. Primary projection, in combination with distortion and denial, eliminates anxiety, but in so doing it impairs the patient's ability to deal with the realities of the world. Secondary projection relieves anxiety to some degree, but the patient retains his ability to deal with realities of the world.

The level of the patient's personality organization has a great deal to do with the use of these defense mechanisms. For example, a primitive character structure where omnipotence and magic predominate and identifications are almost non-existent is associated with primary projection. The patient's inability to establish meaningful interpersonal relations is quite characteristic. He relates to others in a "black and white," "all-or-none" way and tends to view other people only as a source of gratification for himself. This attitude leads to chaos. On the other hand, a patient who uses secondary projection has a more mature personality and his interpersonal relations are more durable.

Two kinds of paranoid symptoms which are encountered clinically may result from these kinds of projections. Paranoid delusions with conviction are associated with primary projection, while mild paranoid ideas with anxiety and doubt are usually encountered with secondary projection and to a greater or lesser degree are seen more commonly.

It should be noted that the presence or absence of another person is of crucial importance to the patient. When he is threatened with loss or abandonment he immediately becomes angry, and his hostility is accompanied by terrifying sadistic fantasies. Being aware of the intensity and unending fury of these fantasies, the patient tries to eliminate them at once and uses projection to do the job. This projected hostility now appears to emanate from another person, whom the patient views as his persecutor while he regards himself as a victim. He may even feel compelled to retaliate in self defense. At such times a homicide may occur. If the persecutor is an individual of the same sex as the patient, he is feared more than a person of the opposite sex. Thus, homosexual paranoid delusions may be viewed clinically as a sign of more serious psychopathology.

These theoretical considerations may be of some significance for the psychotherapy of our patients. Since the decrease of anxiety is the aim of anxiety-suppressive psychotherapy, the therapist must establish rapport with the patient early and maintain it at all costs. With paranoid patients this is a difficult task, but in some cases it can be accomplished paradoxically by encouraging the patient to project his hostile feelings upon the therapist. As it usually happens, the therapist who under-cuts the projections, disclaims responsibility, and avoids associating himself with the patient's suspicions about him, leaves the patient alone to face the intensity of his sadistic fantasies which he is unable to tolerate. By accepting the paranoid attack upon himself, the therapist is able to become involved with the patient and to reassure him. At the same time he becomes the recipient of whatever positive feelings may exist. Since he does not threaten the patient with abandonment, a relationship is possible and it may be established slowly. As a result of this the patient may also accept medication, which, up to this time he usually refuses because of his delusional thoughts about it.

From then on in the same way as a parent handles the realistic fears of his children, the therapist must demonstrate repeatedly that whenever he is threatened with separations, the patient develops his symptoms when he starts to project his anger upon others. At such times his outbursts and aggressive behavior tend to alienate other people from him, and it is then that he becomes confused and experiences anxiety. It is this anxiety that the patient must learn to anticipate. By rehearsing and preparing for such hazards, he may eventually learn to rehabilitate himself.

It should be emphasized, then, that long-term anxiety-suppressive psychotherapy may help some borderline or paranoid patients stay out of mental hospitals and keep intact a good relationship with their dependents. This creates a relatively stable family atmosphere which, in my opinion, plays a crucial role in helping to keep the children emotionally healthy.

5

"CRISIS INTERVENTION"

Assessment of the following factors is necessary in estimating the intensity of an emotional crisis:[1] (1) a history of hazardous situations that led to the development of anxiety; (2) a precipitating event that led to a sudden intensification of the anxiety which gave rise to the emotional crisis; (3) an attempt to cope with this particular anxiety by use of adaptive or maladaptive reactions. The use of these terms, however, implies a certain value judgment on the part of the therapist. Is it possible that what may be considered to be a maladaptive response turns out to be satisfactory as far as the patient is concerned? Certainly, a distinction should be made as to what is accomplished by these reactions. There are several possibilities available. They may serve to deal with, or possibly to eliminate, the anxiety experienced by the patient. They may create a new and at times better emotional equilibrium or help the patient return to the emotional state which existed prior to the development of the emotional crisis. They may give rise temporarily to psychiatric symptoms, they may establish a clear-cut neurosis, or they may finally lead to a psychotic breakdown.

It should be kept in mind, therefore, that the terms "adaptive" and "maladaptive" are used here to denote the therapist's assessment of the patient's solutions. In the same way as a surgeon is alarmed by the refusal of a patient, who has consulted him about a painful abscess in her back, to have a biopsy of a nontender nodule on the breast which has been discovered on physical examination, so is a psychiatrist upset by a patient who, having eliminated his anxiety by various actions, is not further motivated to investigate the reasons for its existence. The following case is given as an illustration.

A twenty-three-year-old soldier, who had just returned from Vietnam, was referred from the dermatology clinic because of neurodermatitis. Having just arrived in Boston, he was in high spirits because he had survived the war and because he was planning to be married to his "only love." At the airport he was greeted by his fiancée, who, it appeared to him, was not very pleased to see him. This worried him, but he decided not to say anything about it just then. During the following week because of various parties and entertainments given in his honor, he did not have time to think much about this disturbing thought. At a dinner party, two days before he came to the skin clinic, his girl friend announced to him that she was pregnant by another man whom she did not love and said she had decided not to see the patient for a while in order to think things over by herself. He was very calm, tried to comfort her, and felt sympathetic and understanding of her difficulties. However, he was unable to sleep during that night and kept thinking somewhat obsessively about what was the "right thing to do."

The next day he was preoccupied with indecision. The thought of adopting the baby or breaking up the relationship with his fiancée bothered him so much that it made him tense. He was in the midst of an emotional crisis. It is of interest that he did not try to assess what role his long absence had to do with his girl friend's predicament.

The next day his skin started to itch, and soon after he developed generalized dermatitis. He was seen by a dermatologist on several occasions. Because he was preoccupied about what to do with his girl friend and because he failed to respond to treatment, he was referred to the psychiatry clinic. When he appeared there he was tense and complained of the itching as well as of vague aches and pains all over his body. He seemed to be passive and dependent and wanted very much to be told how to solve his problem. He asked for advice as to what to do, but when he was encouraged to examine the whole problem he was unwilling to do so and became annoyed.

During the second visit the situation changed. His main preoccupation now was with the dermatitis, which had become worse. He claimed that his mother had solved his problem. She told him that if this skin trouble were to continue he would be unable to get married, anyhow, so it would be preferable to break up with his fiancée and not to have to face the embarrassment of getting married in that condition. Anyway, his mother strongly disapproved of the girl's pregnancy.

After this he felt better and saw no need to continue to come to the psychiatry clinic. He was given another appointment in the hope that he would change his mind, but he did not appear. In a month's time he called to say he was living with his mother, that his skin condition had cleared up completely, and that he had broken off his engagement. The skin disease, irrespective of whether it was psychosomatic or not, served a purpose. It remains to be seen whether it was adaptive or maladaptive.

The patient's history revealed that he was an only child and had always been very close to his mother, and because he had had attacks of asthma when he was very young, she tended to overprotect him. When he was six years old he developed allergies that plagued him for many years. His father was a hard-working man who was never at home because he carried two jobs at the same time in order to support his family. The patient was satisfied to stay at home rather than to play with other children. At times he had serious quarrels with his mother — particularly when she refused his demands. He was a good student, but he had few friends. He did not date except with his fiancée, of whom his mother approved. The mother thought the girl would be a good wife for him. After graduating from high school he was drafted. He was engaged to be married at the time he departed for Vietnam. His army record was excellent. He was not afraid of combat. He spent most of his time alone reading. He never went out with other soldiers and never dated. He wrote to his fiancée three times a week.

Despite the lack of specific details, one may conclude from this cursory summary of this young man's past history that he is potentially vulnerable because he is unable to handle his interpersonal relations in a more mature way. He deals with his emotional crisis by obsessive preoccupation and utilizes his physical symptoms in a way which will enable him to solve his problem. He gets his mother to give him the advice he wants to hear. He rids himself of his fiancée and decides to live with his mother. Although his symptoms have temporarily helped him to overcome his crisis, one may be suspicious as far as his psychodynamic adjustment in the future is concerned. The question that must be raised is: what will happen when this young man is faced in the future with hazardous situations which put a strain on his interpersonal relations? One may speculate that he may develop either psychiatric or physical symptoms. In either event, one would expect him to be passive and expecting to be told what to do. It is also possible, however, that he may be able to adjust well, as he did during his service in the Vietnam war and during his previous twenty years at home. It remains to be seen whether his dependence upon his mother is adequate to help him avert difficulties in the future. What will happen to this man when his mother dies? Will he decompensate at that time, or will he then marry a "motherly" girl who would be willing to satisfy all his demands and thus help him to remain symptom free?

As has been discussed, crisis intervention is specifically aimed at helping an individual overcome his emotional crisis in order to avoid the further development of neurotic difficulties. Its emphasis is basically on prevention. The line of demarcation between evaluation and therapy is not clear cut, and, at times, even one interview may furnish far-reaching psychotherapeutic benefits for the patient. It is important, then, to select individuals who could benefit from crisis intervention, and it should be strongly emphasized that the decision concerning the patient's suitability must be reached as quickly as possible.

Criteria for Selection

The criteria for selection of patients for crisis intervention are essentially similar to those for short-term anxiety-provoking psychotherapy, which will be discussed at length in the following chapter. Here it is sufficient to say that the patients must be in the midst of an emotional crisis, must be intelligent, must give a history of interaction with at least one other person which appears to be meaningful, and must be able to express affect during the evaluation interview. Furthermore, they must be motivated to overcome the emotional crisis, not by magical expectation of help from others but by making efforts to explore and to try to understand, and must show that they have taken active steps in an effort to deal with the crisis. The major emphasis, therefore, should be upon the assessment of these steps — these very reactions which the patient is utilizing.

In general, flexibility is of importance because it denotes the ability of the patient to call upon all kinds of defense mechanisms in an effort to see which appropriate combinations of reactions are best suited to deal with this particular emotional predicament. It should be repeated, however, that the patient is in a state of flux. The therapist should not be particularly disturbed, therefore, if he encounters an individual who uses pathological defense mechanisms — such as projection introjection or denial — as long as these reactions are not used excessively, rigidly, or repetitively. The patient has to call upon all his resources to deal with danger. Obviously the more methods he uses, the more he is able to experiment with different solutions, the better it is.

Requirements and Technique

In the technique of emotional crisis intervention the therapist utilizes the patient's motivation to establish rapport in order to make the therapeutic work a joint venture and transform it as soon as possible into a learning experience. For example, he makes such statements as, "I can try to help you, but you must realize that only you can overcome your problem," or "You must become the surgeon, hold the kinfe, and do the operating. I shall hold your hand." In this way, the prospect of the work to be done is quickly clarified. In addition, the therapist must help the patient to review and understand the steps that led to the development of the emotional crisis itself. Following is an example.

A twenty-eight-year-old newly married man came to the clinic, referred by his family physician, with the diagnosis of tension headache. He claimed that his headache had been present for about two months. It appears that what made him consider seeking medical opinion was a talk he had had with his wife while he was driving her home from her obstetrician's office. At that time his wife had told him of her fears about her impending delivery. He felt apprehensive about this and soon developed a mild headache, which continued, however, despite his taking aspirin. Vague fears about his own health came to his mind. He soon started to think about cancer.

The previous night his wife had gone into labor and had given birth to a seven-pound boy. He had spent all night in the hospital. He was pleased about having a son, but he was not as happy as he had anticipated he would be. After visiting his wife, the thought suddenly occurred to him that his headache might be caused by a brain tumor. He felt frightened and went to see his family doctor, who reassured him and referred him to the psychiatry clinic.

In his interview, he mentioned that he had thought there was a psychological aspect to his problem but was not clear about it. He was motivated "to get to the bottom of this thing."

He was asked again to review the sequence of events which led to his coming to the hospital. Why, for example, did the thought that there might be something seriously wrong with him occur after he visited his wife? How did the thought come to his mind? He answered that it was after thinking that his wife was not as glad to see him as he had expected she would be.

Doctor: Why was that?

Patient: Maybe she was still groggy or in pain.

Doctor: Was she?

Patient: No. She seemed okay.

Doctor: Any other reason?

Patient (hesitating): Maybe she wanted him rather than me.

Doctor: Him?

Patient: You know — the baby.

Doctor: I see! You felt left out?

Patient (somewhat embarrassed): In a way, yes.

Doctor: Have you ever had a feeling like this before?

Patient: Yes. Throughout all this time.

Doctor: What do you mean?

Patient: Lately — you know, all during her pregnancy. Betty was sort of preoccupied.

Doctor: You mean she didn't pay attention to you?

Patient: Yes. You see, she always liked to give me a back rub and stuff like that, but she stopped — I thought at times . . . it sounds crazy . . .

Doctor: Hmm . . . go ahead.

Patient: You know, if I would get sick, Betty would pay attention to me again. She used to give me back rubs, most often when I had a cold, or when I was sick in bed.

Doctor: So being sick would get your wife's attention?
Patient: Yes.
Doctor: How sick?
Patient: You know — sick.
Doctor: No, I don't know.
Patient: Sick, ill, stuff like that.
Doctor: Cancer, maybe?
Patient: . . . Oh, come on. You don't mean this fear of cancer idea has anything to do with all this?
Doctor: I don't know. Does it? What do you think?
Patient: Come to think of it, my wife did talk about cancer that time after her visit to the obstetrician. She had said that at the time of delivery sometimes they discover that women have cancer. I did not give it a thought at the time.
Doctor: But it was then that you developed your headache?
Patient (emphatically): Yes, soon after, but I didn't connect the two.
Doctor: True, but you did yesterday?
Patient: Yes, that's right. It was yesterday that the thought of cancer, or a brain tumor, came to my mind.

Obvious as this case may be, it required systematic work for the details to be amassed during the first interview and the pieces to be put together.

Practical and realistic attempts to solve the emotional crisis should be encouraged. Following is an example.

A twenty-eight-year-old married woman came to the psychiatry clinic in a state of acute anxiety following an ultimatum from her husband, who threatened to divorce her if she did not postpone a visit to her parents. He gave her one week to come to a decision.

It was apparent that this woman had not been able to view her predicament objectively and had not talked to another person about it. She was generally passive in her interview and asked to be told what to do. She was encouraged to make her own decision, and the following week she announced that she had postponed her visit to her parents and had decided to go to New York to think things over. During this time she was able to reconstitute her defenses and make her decisions, all of which helped her to overcome her emotional crisis. One month later she was living with her husband and had her relations with her parents under control.

63

One of the points which has already been discussed emphasizes that while the patient is in the midst of an emotional crisis a golden opportunity is presented to the therapist to intervene before the patient's unsuccessful attempts to deal with his problem give rise to psychiatric symptoms which may eventually crystallize into a neurosis. It must be remembered, however, that once a neurotic symptom has been formed, it may appear to the patient to be the best compromise between the opposing forces of his emotional conflict and may seem to be the best solution to his emotional problem because it alleviates somewhat the anxiety which preceded it. One may even envisage the patient clinging to his symptoms. For it is possible that once psychiatric symptoms are formed, they may become relatively independent of any further psychodynamic interactions, as in a physiological model about learning. In his book *Integrative Activity of the Brain* Konorski, as reported by Gross,[2] theorizes that "kinesthetic gnostic fields" need sensory information for their development, but after they have been formed they remain fairly independent of sensory feedback. If this holds true about psychiatric symptoms, the patient's well-known tendency to resist any interference from the outside which may help him to revert back to his anxious state, may be due to his inability to do anything to change the symptoms themselves. The alternative which is then left to him is to change his attitude about the symptoms and learn to live with them.

Patients at times are almost adamant in their efforts to resist the challenges of their therapists. A young woman put it as follows: "Who do you think you are, to tell *me* how to solve my troubles? I know that you are an expert, but I have found a way out of my misery. It seems that it suits me best, although I am paying a price for it. I am not going to give it up. Your solution may be better, but I am not willing to take a chance." Of course, it should be made explicitly clear to the patient that the therapist does not have any ready-made solutions to offer and that his role is to discuss, to raise questions, and to offer alternatives for the patient to choose from. Even so, explanations sometimes do not help. It is obviously important, therefore, for the therapist to challenge the patient's maladaptive reactions which eventually lead to symptom formation and to try to undercut rigidly fixed solutions of the emotional crisis. Thus, the role of the therapist in crisis intervention is anxiety-provoking.

Following the visit from his mother-in-law, a twenty-five-year-old obese night watchman had a quarrel with his wife, who told him that she would choose her mother over him "any time." As a result of this, he became anxious, and he soon developed a fear of walking in the street. This phobia finally forced him to stop going to work, but it also created an emotional crisis for his wife, who handled the situation by taking matters into her own hands. She had her mother take care of the children while she went out and found a job. This new state of affairs, although not of her choosing, gave her the satisfaction of being the breadwinner of the family. She encouraged her husband to seek psychiatric help. She made the appointments for him at the clinic, which he cancelled, and she finally took time off from work to bring him to the clinic herself. The husband, however, appeared totally unmotivated to give up the phobias which served his passivity, and he actively resisted any plans for psychotherapy. In this sense the phobias which he developed as a way to deal with his emotional crisis appeared to him to be the perfect solution of his emotional problem. Since his wife seemed satisfied in her new role, a new status quo had been established.

The therapist must challenge and minimize the value of actions that he considers to be antitherapeutic and which may lead to further complications. Although the therapist's attitude may be described as authoritarian, faced with the prospect of actions which could lead to serious difficulties for the patient, he, in turn may be forced to act to stop them. The therapist should also try to teach the patient to anticipate situations which are likely to give rise to other emotional difficulties similar to the ones he is experiencing. This educational dimension is an invaluable aspect of crisis intervention. Finally, the crisis intervention should be terminated early in order to avoid characterological entanglements which lead to prolongation of the treatment.

The therapeutic intervention, which was used to help the

woman married to the husband with the borderline personality (Case 3 of Chapter 3), may demonstrate some of the technical details of this procedure. An attempt was made to convince the patient that her husband was still in need of her help, and it was pointed out that she could, if she wanted to, still help him. After all, he was sick, and sick people at times express their anger at the ones they love most. Her husband's anger was presented to her as a symptom of his illness. Divorce or separation, or any other kind of action of this sort which she was considering, would mean abandoning a sick man in need. The therapist finally asked her why her husband's angry feelings created such a need for flight and escape. She responded by describing some of her early experiences with parents in general, and his father in particular, and was able to express, in turn, a great deal of anger at both her parents and her husband in the next two interviews. She soon professed, however, willingness to help him. As her hostility was drained off during the crisis intervention, she was able to understand her own role. She soon announced to her husband that she would not leave him. Although he accepted her statements reluctantly at first, he soon relaxed and was again willing to be taken care of. Despite her wish to continue her visits "in case of trouble," the therapist terminated the treatment.

Crisis intervention not only offered this woman an opportunity to ventilate her hostility toward her husband but also enabled her to understand the nature of her relationship with him. This in turn helped her to evade both the development of psychiatric symptoms and the flight which she contemplated. As the belief that she was essential to him was reinforced, she was able to mobilize her resources quickly and to reestablish her emotional equilibrium.

It could be argued that this woman needed long-term psychotherapy to alter her masochistic behavior. This is silly. A point has been reached when this patient again was willing to help nurse her husband as she had done in the past and this, in turn, contributed to his becoming stabilized. Enough is enough.

A special aspect of crisis intervention involves helping young mothers deal with emotional crises which result from their relations with their children.[3] Child psychiatrists know a great deal about this kind of problem, but they generally tend to deal with such situations with the well-known standardized approach, namely, the child psychiatrist treats the child and the social worker treats the mother. In my opinion, it is possible for one to intervene and help the mother resolve her emotional crisis without necessarily assuming that the child must also be treated. Actually, the child's behavior may be followed by outside observers and may become an independent indicator of the mother's progress in the resolution of her emotional crisis.

A thirty-one-year-old mother of three children came to a mental health agency with her six-year-old son, referred by his teacher because "of an unusually docile behavior at school." He appeared withdrawn from other children, tense, and he constantly bit his fingernails. In direct contrast was his behavior at home, where he was aggressive with both his mother and his siblings. The boy was the oldest of three. He had no feeding problems, had walked and talked at a normal age, and was toilet trained by the end of eighteen months without difficulty. He had not seemed to be disturbed by the birth of his siblings and had been in good physical health. In sum, he had an essentially normal development.

According to his mother, he became dependent upon her when he was five years old and soon began to react with unusual anger when she would not give in to his demands. She emphasized that she had always had a strong desire to be independent herself and added that she also taught her children to be independent. It appeared that both she and her husband had put pressure on the oldest boy to do good work at school, even when he was in the first grade, and he had responded by working hard. Although they had continued to praise him, his ferocity seemed to continue unabated when his demands were not satisfied by his mother. The boy spoke often about violent deaths, and when, on one occasion, he hit one of his brothers on the head, causing some bleeding, for which he was punished severely by his mother, he reacted with a temper tantrum.

The boy was seen by the child psychiatrist of the agency and was also observed on two occasions while at school. There he did not partake in the class discussion and did not communicate with other children during the study hour. When asked questions, however, he always came out with the correct answer, and seemed to be interested and alert when the teacher paid attention to him. During recess he would run — or, rather, gallop — aimlessly along, all alone, over the playground until, finally exhausted, he would sit down by himself. It was the child psychiatrist's impression that although he appeared somewhat shy, he seemed to be a fairly normal boy with no ascertainable serious emotional disturbance.

The father also was interviewed at the agency. He drew essentially the same picture of the boy as the mother had done but emphasized that his wife had great expectations of their son and pushed him intensively to achieve success. It appeared that the mother's excessive need for independence might play a role in her child's behavior, and she was asked to come back to be interviewed by the psychiatrist. It developed that she was the oldest of four girls. Her father was a heavy drinker and was unable to support the family. The mother had to go out to work, and at a very early age she, herself, was given a great deal of responsibility in running the household and bringing up her sisters. She resented all this bitterly, but, being a perfectionist, she met those challenges well. Although willing and capable, she could not go to college. She was married when she was young and successfully managed her family, including her husband, with an iron hand. She was seen in crisis intervention six times. The main focus of the work centered around the "problem of her son." At first she was hesitant to give information about herself: "After all, I came here to talk about my son's problems," she said. She soon relaxed, however, and discussed her life fully and easily. She described with much emotion her anger against her father and her subsequent feeling of guilt. She also talked about her mixed feelings regarding her mother. When she realized that she was treating her son in the same way that her parents had treated her — in a manner she thought very unfair, she became less demanding of him. Having talked freely about her hostile feelings toward her sisters, she was able to realize that her older son might also harbor angry feelings and jealousy for his own younger siblings. She could also see that his negativistic behavior toward her when she failed to gratify his wishes was a way for him to express his own need for rebellion. As she became more understanding, she was soon able to give the boy special privileges as the oldest son and arranged for special times which he and she could share together. She did all this without hesitation. As time went by, her anxiety subsided. She was more tolerant of her son and more at ease with him. After she visited her parents for the first time in six years, she announced with pride that she felt very little tension when she was with them — something that had not ever happened before.

The boy, also, responded rapidly to the change in his mother. His aggressive behavior at home practically disappeared as he became more cooperative. He again started to play with his siblings and with other boys in the neighborhood without getting into fights. At school his behavior was less tense and withdrawn.

As the mother became more self-confident, she began to talk about how much she enjoyed her son's improved behavior, and added, "Now I am able to understand his problems."

Another example of successful intervention with the mother follows.

A five-year-old-boy and his mother were referred to the mental health agency by their pediatrician because of the boy's fear of being injured. The child psychiatrist who saw the boy decided that it was not necessary to offer therapy at the time. However, he thought that the boy should be seen occasionally because it was possible that if his phobia did not clear up, he might require treatment in the future.

The mother had six interviews over a period of two months. She gave the following history: The boy was her first child. She had been unhappy about her pregnancy and had experienced a difficult delivery. The baby had had no feeding problems, had the usual childhood diseases, and had developed normally up to about six months before she came to the agency. It was during the summer and while the boy was playing on the beach that he saw one of his friends who had broken his leg and was wearing a cast. He seemed to be unusually interested in his friend's misfortune. He was told by his mother that "bad boys who misbehave sometimes fall down and break their legs." He appeared to pay little attention to that statement at the time. Five months later, while he was playing with a ball in their yard, the ball rolled outside the fence. As he ran out to catch it a car sped by. His mother, who was running after him, was very upset and gave him a spanking. She told him that he should be careful because the car would have "hit him and cut his leg off." Following this episode the boy became upset, was unable to sleep, had occasional nightmares, and asked for constant reassurance from his mother about not losing his leg and not being injured. It was then that the mother remembered about the episode on the beach, grew alarmed, and took her son to their pediatrician, who referred them both to the mental health agency.

The mother was thirty-five years old. An only child, she had been brought up by two rigid parents who had been divorced when she was twelve. From then on, she lived with her father, whom she described as "very sadistic," and who, when under the influence of alcohol, enjoyed undressing her and slapping her repeatedly on the face. After she had graduated from high school, she worked as a secretary for twelve years under a very authoritarian man and then married her husband, whom she described as being somewhat passive. She was dissatisfied with her married life and always had the desire to return to work. Unhappy in her domestic role, she tried to adjust to it by taking meticulous care of her son and of her household. She admitted to being frustrated and angry at times and described herself as a domineering mother and wife.

She related fairly well but had a tendency to try to dominate the interviewer. She was an intelligent woman, who was willing to question her role as a mother and the possibility that she may have contributed in precipitating her son's phobia. When it became clear to her that, at certain periods of development, children in general and boys in particular may become quite attached or dependent upon their mothers, she mentioned that she had noticed that her son had been especially attached to her over the last year. She admitted that she had occasionally been embarrassed by his affectionate caresses and realized that her threats of punishment were due in part to her uneasiness about this. She thought she might have been a bit too harsh with him. An effort was made to associate her hostility and her resentment of her father's domination over her with her own tendency to dominate her passive husband and her male child. As her own role became clear to her she reported that she had tried to be more lenient, had stopped her threats, and had responded to her son's playfulness. She was encouraged to continue and appeared to be more relaxed. In the last interview, she reported that the boy had no more disturbing dreams, had stopped complaining about his phobic symptoms, and did not seek constant reassurance. She said she was very encouraged. One year later, when her son entered the first grade, she reported that he seemed to be doing very well and had many friends. His phobias had not returned. She was pleased with the progress and felt she had contributed to it.

People who experience life as being frightening tend to become sick. Crisis intervention is a way to help them make the world appear less threatening.

Anxiety-provoking psychotherapy is offered to individuals who have considerable strength of character but, while facing hazardous situations and as a result of being unable to overcome their emotional crises, have developed circumscribed psychiatric symptoms and/or difficulties in their interpersonal relations. This kind of treatment is similar in theory to psychoanalytic or psychodynamic psychotherapy. As we have seen already, an area of emotional conflict underlying the patient's interpersonal difficulties or symptoms or both is defined jointly as the patient's emotional problem, which is to be solved during the therapy. The patient is motivated, but he is also encouraged by his therapist to work through his difficulties. Furthermore, he is able to tolerate a certain degree of anxiety which is generated during the interview by the therapist's anxiety-provoking questions. These are intended to stimulate the patient to explore and understand his emotional problem and its underlying conflicts. When the patient experiences the emotions involved in them during the interview and recognizes the reactions which he utilizes, he has finally learned to resolve his difficulties. Crisis intervention lasts up to two months, and short-term anxiety-provoking psychotherapy lasts anywhere from two to twelve months, with an average of about three to five months. These time intervals are not rigid, however. Psychoanalysis, of course, is anxiety-provoking psychotherapy of long-term duration.

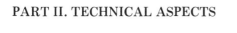

PART II. TECHNICAL ASPECTS

6

SELECTION OF PATIENTS

Selection of appropriate patients for short-term anxiety-provoking psychotherapy is essential. It involves both the careful assessment of each patient's psychodynamics and the fulfillment of five specific selection criteria.

The evaluation of the patient's psychodynamics, as already mentioned, involves setting up a tentative hypothesis and arriving at a formulation based on the detailed information which has been obtained from the patient during the history-taking of his emotional development. As a result of this, certain ideas are formed in the evaluator's mind about the emotional conflicts underlying the patient's interpersonal difficulties and symptoms, or both, which may help to explain his overall behavioral patterns. These ideas must then be explored at length in the interview. No idle speculation should be allowed. Just as the gifted clinician has amassed a whole array of important details as he goes through the process of the differential diagnosis of a complaint of pain in the chest and proceeds systematically to collect appropriate information from the patient and to rule out various diseases until he is certain of the correct diagnosis, so must the psychiatrist obtain specific information from the patient to confirm and substantiate his psychodynamic formulation. Furthermore, because he cannot rely on laboratory tests to confirm his diagnosis, he must depend entirely upon the tangible evidence which the patient, and only the patient, can reveal to him.

The psychodynamic formulation then becomes the solid foundation upon which the whole therapeutic structure is going to be built. It is similar to the knowledge of anatomy which guides the surgeon in the performance of a complicated operation. As the surgeon may expect anatomical variations and be prepared to change his technical approach to deal with them, so must the psychiatrist be ready to alter his formulation in the light of new evidence which is uncovered during the course of the therapy. But more about this later.

In the psychiatry clinic of the Massachusetts General Hospital, between the years 1954 and 1968, we saw many patients who seemed to be good candidates for short-term anxiety-provoking psychotherapy. It became necessary for us, therefore, to set up specific criteria to use in the selection of such patients from the great number of individuals who were seeking psychiatric help. It should be emphasized that some of their complaints, compared with the severity of the symptoms of others, may appear trivial at first glance. On closer scrutiny, however, it becomes clear that these problems not only were very incapacitating to the patients but also created difficulties in their everyday lives, restricted their freedom, interfered seriously with their future potential, and finally radiated distress to several key members of their immediate environment.

The Clinic Setting

The psychiatry clinic patient population during these years was composed largely of young people ranging in age from seventeen to forty-five. Many were students in the various colleges and universities of the greater Boston area, while others were recent graduates of these same schools. There was a small percentage of patients who came from more distant places, who had gone out of their way and had taken consider-able trouble to commute to the hospital.

Many came on their own initiative, while others arrived following the recommendation of ex-patients who had found their experience in the clinic to be helpful. Several were referred from psychiatrists in the various university health services. When it became well known that we were specializing in short-term psychotherapy, the clinic population increased rapidly, yet because of the shorter time interval required for treatment more time was made available to the therapists to see more patients.

This kind of psychotherapy was conducted by advanced residents in psychiatry or young junior staff psychiatrists who had learned the technique we utilized by treating several patients as a part of their training under my personal supervision. A seminar involving a continuous case presentation of short-term anxiety-provoking psychotherapy was held every year from 1960 through 1967 and was attended by all the residents assigned to the clinic, the student social workers, several staff social workers, as well as by a group of Harvard medical students on occasions.

We used five admission evaluating teams, with a different senior resident in charge for each day of the week, to evaluate all patients coming to the clinic.[1] The participating members of each team included junior residents in psychiatry, staff social workers, social work and medical students, as well as occasionally community mental health fellows, psychologists, and social scientists.

Those patients who were considered to be appropriate candidates for short-term anxiety-provoking psychotherapy by these various "teams" were seen in an administrative goal-setting interview. Certain guidelines were set during this interview regarding the length of treatment. These patients were told that they had been selected to receive a treatment in which the clinic specialized, which was going to last a few months only. No rigid time limits were set. In addition, during this interview an attempt was made to reevaluate the selection criteria and particularly the patient's motivation for psychotherapy. Certain predictions were also made of what to expect during the process of psychotherapy and of what its outcome was going to be.

After spending considerable time in reviewing records, interviewing patients as well as their therapists, and looking

77

over psychotherapy notes, we finally were able to develop the following criteria, which we used as guidelines for the evaluation and selection of our patients.[2]

Selection Criteria

1. The patient must be of above-average intelligence.

An effort was made to assess intelligence by obtaining adequate information about the patient's exceptional work performance or superior academic and other educational achievements, and not to rely on psychological testing. The ability to conceptualize and even intellectualize, contrary to the generally held notion that it can be used as a resistance, facilitated, if anything, the psychotherapeutic work; for there is a cognitive, as well as an emotional dimension, to short-term anxiety-provoking psychotherapy. Problem-solving requires intelligence, and the more intelligent one is the better he solves his problems. On the rare occasions when psychological tests were used, the interviewer's rating of a patient's intelligence was not far off from his actual I. Q.

2. The patient must have had at least one meaningful relationship with another person during his lifetime.

One should define the word "meaningful." It implies shared intimacy, emotional involvement, trust, and also an ability to give and take. The way in which one human being relates with another is the *ultimate* test of his ability to deal with the realities of everyday life. The difference between the expected stability of material objects compared with the unpredictable responses and fickle inconsistencies of human behavior requires forbearance and tolerance. The patient who has had one such relationship has the ability to withstand anxiety, and this should indicate his having developed a fairly mature personality. On the other hand, if he has had no such experience, this should alert the evaluator to the probability that he is dealing with someone who would not be able to relate to the therapist during treatment and would look upon it only as a source of gratification. The way to assess this criterion is not to accept at face value the patient's statement about his having had good relations but to question him extensively about the nature of these relationships. Information about participation in group membership, such as work, family, and club, may give an overall picture; and such questions as "What did you do for him? Did you sacrifice anything for his sake? Is your friendship continuing at the present time? How often do you see each other"? may give the evaluator considerable and specific information about interpersonal relations.

What is necessary is to establish that the patient is able to be altruistic or at least is capable of reciprocating. For example, a patient may claim to have had many friends, yet, upon close questioning, it soon becomes apparent that all these so-called friendships are basically used as sources of gratification, in which the patient's own interests always come first, compared with the needs of someone else. Thus, except for providing satisfaction to the patient, such relationships are essentially meaningless. An example follows.

A single, thirty-two-year-old artist said that his best friend was his college roommate and insisted that their friendship had not changed over the years. They saw each other, however, only during college reunions, although they lived only three miles apart. When the patient was asked to give an example about the nature of their friendship he announced, "Well, I was good in sports those days and my roommate always used to build me up. He would come and tell me all the good things the coach and other kids had to say about my performance." When the interviewer asked what he did to reciprocate, the patient looked puzzled and said, "What was there for me to do? I told you that he was my best friend. He made me happy. Isn't that enough? My painting does this for me nowadays, better than anything else." Such a statement is revealing, in that art to this individual is more satisfying than human interactions.

The assessment of a meaningful relationship in the patient's past history does not necessarily have to involve a member of his immediate family. There are individuals who appear to have been totally devoid of human contacts in the past yet appear to be fairly well adjusted in the present. Persistent scrutiny and review of interpersonal relations will almost invariably reveal a meaningful contact which, at first glance, had been obscured and was not obvious. Following is an example.

An eighteen-year-old college freshman came to the clinic because of depression after his girl friend died of leukemia. His mother was an alcoholic, and his father divorced her when the patient was only a few months old. He was brought up by his paternal grandmother, whom he hated because she was tyrannical. His father, an army man, was "never at home" and seemed to prefer his sister, who was eight years his senior. His grandmother had a maid, an elderly spinster who, as things turned out, was the person who actually brought him up, spent all her free time with him, and occasionally had affectionately called him the child she never had. She died when he was eight years old. He was heartbroken, and ever since then he had suppressed the importance of this relationship with her. It was from that time that his grandmother took over his upbringing and started her strict punishing ways; but those eight years with his grandmother's maid gave him a warm human contact, made a significant difference in his upbringing, and helped him develop the security of human relations which he utilized advantageously during the following years.

3. The patient must be able to interact with the evaluating psychiatrist by expressing appropriately some feeling during the interview and showing some degree of flexibility.

The patient's ability to interact meaningfully with another person may require verification. The interviewer has a golden opportunity to make this test during the interview by assessing the way in which the patient interacts with him. The appropriate expression of emotion during the interview, of course, demonstrates that the patient has access to his feelings, which do not necessarily have to be positive ones. A patient who is aware, for example, of his anger, sadness, fear, or his joy and affection, and is able to express openly such feelings during the interview shows that he is in control of these emotions and is not frightened by them. If, for example, as a result of the history-taking, the patient gets angry because of a question from the interviewer and is able to deal with this emotion, acknowledge it, and express it appropriately, he is considered a better candidate than someone who covers up his reaction and tries to be ingratiating rather than truthful.

The expression of emotion has to be assessed quantitatively and qualitatively, for it should be remembered that schizophrenic patients who are notorious for having "a lack of affect" can at times have violent emotional explosions which they may express murderously. The ability, then, not only to recognize and express emotions but also to verbalize them is significant. Some patients experience a difficulty in this area.[3] When they are asked to talk about how they feel they mention repetitively and endlessly only somatic sensations, without being able to relate them to any accompanying thoughts, fantasies, or conflicts. Others seem to be unable to specify what it feels like to be angry or sad, and a few individuals fail to differentiate between pleasant and unpleasant emotions. They usually respond to such questioning by describing the actions they take under those circumstances and, when pressed for further details, show irritability and annoyance. Such patients seem to have limited vocabularies. They seem to have marked difficulty in finding appropriate words to describe their emotions. They usually look puzzled and give the impression they do not understand the meaning of the word "feeling." Because of these limitations, such patients tend to have difficulty in communicating with other people and appear to be uninteresting and dull. The interviewer, in turn, experienced in dealing with elaborate verbal communications of ordinary neurotic people, finds it difficult to evaluate such boring patients. Furthermore, because he is unable to make a psychodynamic formulation or to fit the patient into a familiar diagnostic category, he tries to explain away the patient's difficulties by statements such as, "He seems to be denying his feeling."

I would like to introduce the term alexithymic (Greek *a*, lack, *lexis*, word, *thymos*, mood) to describe patients who present these difficulties. What is of interest is that during the evaluation interviews with them, a compromise is usually reached when finally the psychiatrist is forced to talk about the emotions of the patient by providing his own appropriate words to describe them. The patient, in turn, borrows these words gratefully, and by imitating, he parrots them back to his doctor without understanding their real meaning. Usually an impasse is reached. Some patients with psychosomatic illnesses fall into this category. They are not good candidates for short-term anxiety-provoking psychotherapy, and the question must be raised as to the contraindication of psychotherapy in general, which relies so much on verbal and emotional interactions, for such patients. What is the alternative? I have none, but I also feel strongly that psychotherapy should not be used for lack of something better. Research in this area may provide us with a better treatment.

Violent emotions may be sometimes present in patients suffering from ulcerative colitis, but this seems to be the exception rather than the rule.[4] Here is an example of an interview with a twenty-seven-year-old girl suffering from this disease, who seemed to show complete lack of affect during the interview.

The patient's voice was monotonous. She talked about her aunt, who had repeatedly borrowed large sums of money from her and refused to pay her back. The interviewer asked how she felt about this situation. The patient looked puzzled and said that she did not like it.

Doctor: How did you feel?

Patient: I . . . you know, I wanted to hit her over the head.

Doctor: I did not mean what you wanted to do. I wondered how you felt.

Patient (silent for a while): I don't know what you mean.

Doctor: Did you feel angry?

Patient: I guess so.

Doctor: What is it like to feel angry?

Patient: You know, don't you?

Doctor: What does it feel like to you?

Patient: I don't know. There are no words to describe it.

In contrast to such patients, our patients were able to verbalize well and to show a considerable degree of flexibility. Evidence of flexibility, which implies a willingness to see not only one's own but also the other person's side of the conflict, is an important dimension for this criterion, because it gives a clear picture of the ways in which the patient handles his feelings during the interview. Statements such as "I know that my problems with my family have a lot to do with the anger that I feel against my roommate, but there are still many irritating little things that he does which are quite realistic and which annoy me no end,'' denote a degree of flexibility.

At times it may be helpful to have the patient see an interviewer of the same or opposite sex if it is difficult to assess his ability to interact during the questioning. Sometimes such things as unusual hostility and nervousness or exaggerated willingness to please must be assessed on that basis. A patient who had been unusually seductive to both a female medical student and a social worker and talked explicitly to them about his sexual exploits and conquests of women confessed to having acted this role to embarrass them. He admitted to the male interviewing psychiatrist that he disliked women and that he was an overt homosexual.

4. The patient must be able to voice a specific chief complaint.

The ability to circumscribe his complaints denotes freedom of choice which may be viewed as strength of character. The patient is asked to assign top priority to the *one* problem he wants to solve. The clear-cut selection of a specific interpersonal difficulty or a clear-cut symptom chosen from a variety of difficulties usually indicates a fairly stable equilibrium of emotional forces which the patient has at his disposal. The ability to postpone the alleviation of other complaints and the willingness to be forced to select only one shows the patient's potential to withstand stress.

The universal tendency to avoid diffuse anxiety associated with the frightening, alien, strange, or unknown and the search for the familiar, usual, and concrete is well known. A common phenomenon encountered in tourists who visit a foreign country for the first time and who, despite their professed interest in exploration or adventure, tend to associate only with their own countrymen, look shocked and complain about everything which is odd and unfamiliar, talk endlessly about the superiority of their own country or home state and ask for the proverbial "hamburger in Paris," is an example of this tendency. Patients who enter a hospital for the first time cling to their possessions, such as their eyeglasses, not only to explore this new environment but also because the glasses may be the only familiar possession in the midst of a potentially hostile environment. When the glasses are taken away from them they feel estranged and apprehensive. A similar behavior is often observed in patients who suffer from eye diseases and who become totally disoriented when a black patch is placed over their eyes before surgery.

The question must be raised whether, by a different rearing of children or another educational system, we can help people to become more comfortable with the unfamiliar and the unknown and to learn to live with anxiety without development of psychiatric symptoms. If this ever becomes possible, we may be able to bring up children who have the courage to explore and whose minds will expand, not through the medium of drugs or other artificial stimulants, but as a result of their own potentials. This, also, could mark the end of parochial, naive, and rigid behavior patterns which produce "the apathetic connoisseurs of bland clichés, and narrow-minded experts of the obvious detail." If psychotheraphy can help even in a small way in this direction it will have demonstrated its *raison d'être*.

Defense mechanisms, such as displacement, projection, and isolation, help to change a state of diffuse anxiety and bring it under control by producing a concrete, clear-cut, specific symptom — a phobia. The kinds of specific chief complaints which we have encountered most often include such symptoms as anxieties, depressions, phobias, conversions, and mild obsessive-compulsive or behavior and personality disorders involving clear-cut interpersonal difficulties.

5. The patient must be motivated for change, not only for symptom relief, and he must be willing to work hard during his treatment.

Motivation for psychotherapy is possibly the most crucial criterion, because, when we asked patients what was the most important contributing factor in the success of their treatment, they said it was their original willingness to understand themselves. Having been impressed by this finding, we decided to set up specific criteria for evaluation of the patients' motivations for psychotherapy.

Evaluation Criteria for Motivation for Psychotherapy

1. An ability to recognize that the symptoms are psychological

Such an awareness demonstrates a certain degree of psychological sophistication, in contrast with the more common attitude of denial of emotional difficulties, often accompanied by the insistence that the only reason for seeing a psychiatrist is because of the recommendation of the referring physician. An example is the case of a thirty-five-year-old garage mechanic, father of two children, who said, "I thought that my headaches were due to some physical cause. I was angry when the nerve clinic made an appointment for me to see a psychiatrist. When the doctor explained to me that nervousness can aggravate headaches, I realized that when I was tense my headaches became worse. I know that I am nervous, but I did not put the two together."

2. A tendency to be introspective and to give an honest and truthful account of emotional difficulties

A thirty-eight-year-old woman described it this way: "For a long time I had tried to understand why I get scared when I go shopping downtown. I know there is nothing that could happen to me; but as soon as I get out of my car and start walking in the parking lot, my heart begins to pound and my hands start to shake. I have tried having a drink before I go out shopping, but it doesn't help. Then my doctor gave me tranquilizers, but they didn't help, either. I have taken my children along with me, and my girl friend, but nothing works. I am willing to try anything, and I shall endeavor to be as honest as I can in my treatment."

3. Willingness to participate actively in the treatment situation

The implication here is that the patient does not want to be a passive participant but is actively trying to understand his predicament. A twenty-two-year-old girl described how, after each date, she was unable to sleep. "I lie in bed, tossing back and forth, and I keep thinking about my date, the way he looked, the way he danced, and the girls he talked with. I feel quite jealous. I finally get exhausted trying to figure everything out, and I fall asleep. I notice that I feel worse when I am at a cocktail party, so lately I have not been going out." Further-more, such statements as these made by patients: "I do want to understand myself, but I need the doctor to guide me," or "I do not expect to change completely, but I do hope to know myself better as a result of the treatment," show the patient's willingness to work in psychotherapy. In contrast, other patients want to be told exactly what to do: "I am in your hands, doctor" or "I have placed myself in the care of the clinic, and I expect you to tell me what to do." "Am I right in thinking the way I do?" said a passive twenty-one-year-old; and when the doctor stated that she was putting him in the role of a judge or a clergyman, she angrily retorted, "Of course I do. My priest tells me what to do and so does my mother. But it isn't enough. I want everyone to guide me because I am so confused I cannot think straight. After all, I cannot be with my mother and my priest all the time. I expect you to work for me. Isn't it your job"?

4. Curiosity and willingness to understand oneself

Idle curiosity denotes a passive expectation of gratification from another person, but active curiosity may signify self-inquisitiveness, introspection, and a willingness to understand oneself. This latter aspect of curiosity may indicate a motivating trait that can be utilized constructively in psychotherapy.

5. Willingness to change, explore, and experiment

These attitudes seem to be the result of active and construc-tive curiosity on the part of the patient. They reveal some degree of flexibility and show that turning to psychotherapy as an experiment is indicative of a desire to try in a new way to deal with his problem. A twenty-year-old man, complaining of impotence, said, "I must work hard to understand this problem. My family doctor said that it was all in my mind. I know it is in my mind, but it is up to me to figure it out. I am tired of it and I'm prepared to try to do something construc-tively because I want to change."

6. Expectations of the results of psychotherapy

A distinction should be made between unrealistic and realistic expectations. Unrealistic expectations may be vague, wide in scope, nonspecific, exaggerated, and magical. They seem to be the remnants of childhood wish-fulfillment fantasies, omni-potent in nature, which give the indication of a poor assessment of reality. One patient who had never written or published anything came to the clinic expecting that, as a result of the treatment, he would be able to write a novel and win the Pulitzer Prize. Realistic expectations, on the other hand, are usually modest, specific, and circumscribed. "I have talked with you about my worries, about my poor grades, my problems with my father, and my feelings of guilt," said a twenty-year-old single student. "I don't know why, but at the present time I am mad at my roommate. This makes my life miserable. Of course, I could move out of our apartment. However, this would not explain what makes me angry at him. If psychotherapy can make me realize what lies behind these angry outbursts of mine I would be quite satisfied."

7. Willingness to make reasonable sacrifices

Most patients are usually willing to make compromises, but occasionally a seemingly well-motivated patient may prove to be without motivation when he is asked to make a specific sacrifice, such as getting an extra job to pay for psychotherapy or changing his schedule to meet clinic appointments. It may soon become obvious that what was earlier believed to be motivation is dwindling. The patient appears to expect a bargain, wants everything to be arranged to suit him, and is not willing to compromise.

Patients who fulfilled all seven criteria were considered to have had good to excellent motivation, six out of seven to have had fair to good motivation, and four out of seven to have had questionable motivation. All those who fulfilled less than the four criteria were considered to have had poor or no motiva-tion.

For example, we have considered as therapeutic successes only those patients who said that they felt better and whose therapists had also stated that they had improved. Therapeutic failures, on the other hand, involved lack of progress in therapy as viewed by both patient and therapist. Patients who terminated the treatment on their own initiative were considered as failures, even if their therapists thought that some progress had taken place. Our observations tended to show the important role that motivation for psychotherapy plays and also seemed to indicate that patients who show good motivation at the time of selection usually do well in psychotherapy of short duration, while those who are not so motivated do not.

The word "motivation" is not synonymous with the word "cause." Nevertheless, it appears to be a force within an individual that leads to action, and, as such, it is a force that has been extensively studied by psychologists and psychiatrists.[5] Silverman,[6] who reviewed the pertinent work going on regarding motivation for psychotherapy, mentioned several factors that play important roles, such as the patient's suffering and discomfort, his readiness for treatment, his wish for recovery, and his secondary gains. Having considered the subject from a detailed dynamic standpoint, he stresses the conviction that the assessment of overall motivation should be an important factor in pretreatment evaluation work-up.

Although motivational forms seem to be essentially the same,[7] they are handled differently by each individual. From our experience, motivation is defined as "a problem-solving process." It seems to be an all-inclusive kind of stimulus that gives rise to a set of fantasies and thoughts and leads finally to actions which have the specific aim of avoiding the painful feelings of anxiety, frustration, loneliness, and boredom. Thus, such feelings appear to be the very source of this process. Painful feelings of hopelessness and helplessness, on the other hand, are so intense that they cease to be motivational forces and lead only to despair. The motivational actions vary from person to person, but they usually reduce the painful feelings and give rise to a great deal of satisfaction. The pleasurable experience which results from this problem-solving process interestingly enough sets into motion further motivational explorations in order to obtain still greater gratification. Curiosity, which is one of our criteria for assessing motivation regarding psychotherapy, seems to play an important part in this problem-solving pain-pleasure cycle. The motivational process, therefore, can also be viewed as a series of balanced states between painful and pleasurable feelings, rather than as a simple static reflex-like avoidance of pain. As long as the pain is not intense, as mentioned before, and feelings of helplessness and hopelessness are not present, the motivational process will go on.

In addition to curiosity, there is an element of self-entertainment in the motivational process, particularly at times of loneliness and boredom. For it should not be forgotten that we are alone with our own fantasies and thoughts for the major part of our lives. Loneliness is experienced only by those who have never learned to live with themselves but rely on outsiders to provide them with entertainment. Faced with the void inside, and aware of their boredom, they rely on reflex-like actions to fill this vacuum, not realizing the magnificent possibilities of an unexplored world existing within themselves. Such experiences may have their origin in early childhood, possibly when the very young child is left alone in his crib. A patient of mine gave the following description:

When I am faced with an unresolved problem, I start quoting nursery stories. It is a plea for help when I feel unhappy, confused, and lonely. I seek some direction, but I don't get it. I am left all alone. Nursery poems cheer me up, comfort me when I am bored, puzzled, scared, and alone. It is a refuge for me. I used to be lonely and scared in my crib. I cried. I screamed. But after a while I started to look around to explore. Soon I felt better, and I remember trying to think of new nursery rhymes, maybe think of new stories or of new ways to tell the stories that have never been told before — ways that would make me even happier. As I grew up I became a good student in school because I used what I had learned about myself in other situations. Even now, daydreams make me discover myself. I feel so involved in them that a great deal of time passes by. All my worries have disappeared, as well as my fears. All my problems have gone. I am satisfied with myself.

His frustrations led to powerful motivational processes that solved his problems. They were his first steps toward self-understanding. This vivid picture speaks for itself.

Motivation for psychotherapy is also a problem-solving process. The patient who visits a psychiatrist may appear only to want to relieve his discomfort, but soon he is helped to become aware that there may be other ways of dealing with his problem. Thus, he may be willing to change his original expectations, having been excited by his own curiosity to explore himself and to obtain a thorough understanding of his life experiences. The motivational process for psycho-therapy must be encouraged to develop, therefore, and must be reinforced by the outside world. It must be assessed on the basis of the kind of psychotherapy most appropriate for the patient's needs, as has already been mentioned. When no motivation for psychotherapy is evident, it should indicate an absence of painful feelings and subsequent gratifications. This may present a serious problem. Patients who make manipula-tive suicide attempts are usually unmotivated because they derive satisfaction from the use of their morbid manipulative solutions in their interpersonal relationships. The way to motivate them is to find an area that caused them to become anxious and concentrate upon that. Through this approach the motivational process may effect a firm hold upon such patients.

Finally, the motivational process is also associated with the creative process — with its passive and active components. The huge wealth of experiences, fantasies, images, and thoughts which is available to everybody is the passive source from which a motivated individual, with his curiosity, willing-ness to explore, to experiment, and to change, can set in motion the selective processes which transform this static picture into a dynamic one. By choosing appropriate fragments from this vast source, curiosity and motivation again play crucial roles. Satisfaction and restlessness during the selective process, which requires total absorption of the individual for creative work, finally lead to the synthetic process, which deals with assembling seemingly unrelated fragments and components, and synthesizes them into a meaningful whole. This process involves the discovery of hidden similarities or the tolerance of paradoxical situations. All these three aspects of the creative process have to do with inspiration, discovery, and invention.

There is another dimension of creativity that involves the form of its expression. Here talent, painstaking preparation, and hard work are vitally important and are responsible for the final conquering of the artistic medium or the scientific method that play such effective roles in producing a new discovery.[8] Thus, creativity and motivation go hand in hand.

Jean Paul Sartre put it this way in his autobiography, *The Words:*[9]

> Everything took place in my head. Imaginary child that I was, I defended myself with my imagination. When I examine my life from six to nine, I am struck by the continuity of my spiritual exercises. Their content often changed, but the program remained unvaried (page 113).
>
> I would let myself daydream; I would discover, in a state anguish ghastly possibilities, a monstrous universe that was only the underside of my omnipotence. I would say to myself: anything can happen! and that meant: I can imagine anything (page 148).

The motivational process, whether in psychotherapy, in science, or in art, can play a crucial role in making life more exciting.

It should be emphasized, finally, that despite all the selection criteria and despite the extensive evaluation, one should keep an open mind, because he may discover the seriousness of certain well-hidden traits in the patient's character only after psychotherapy has begun. Following is an example.

A thirty-five-year-old married banker developed anxiety when his superior officer talked with him about the prospect of his becoming a vice president. Although he wanted to please him and accept the offer, he felt contented with his present job and did not want any more responsibility. This characteristic of always trying to please people in authority dated back to his relationship with his own father. He liked to view himself as a "good boy," and mentioned that as an adolescent he had developed syphilophobia without ever having had sexual intercourse. He remembered that his mother had reassured him about this, but cautioned him not to talk to his father about it. He was fairly happy in his marriage but was always uneasy about sexual relations, which he tried to avoid whenever possible. This seemingly passive trait was considered ominous, but, because he fulfilled our criteria and seemed to be functioning reasonably well, he was accepted for treatment. In his second interview he announced that another man had been made the vice president of the bank, and he claimed that his anxiety had disappeared. From then on, in his interviews he talked only about pleasant memories, such as "basking in the sun during his vacation." His passivity had been underestimated during the evaluation and, as soon as his anxiety disappeared, the motivation to understand himself vanished. He developed no self-understanding.

During the assessment of the selection criteria, differences of opinion usually arise when one attempts to evaluate some of these difficult points. It is because of this that the system of using the evaluating teams to deal with all new patients has been so helpful. When evaluators have the opportunity to compare and contrast their impressions they eventually arrive at a consensus of opinion about a psychodynamic formulation which helps in understanding the emotional difficulties of a patient.

7

TECHNIQUE

The Therapist and the Patient Face to Face

As there is much divergence of opinion about the whole
subject of psychotherapy, so there is considerable controversy
about the question of technique. For example, at one extreme
there are those who think that no greater sophistication than
common sense is required to sit down and talk with a patient.
They believe that the training of psychiatry residents under
supervision is a waste of time. On the other hand, there are
those who think that every movement, look, gesture, posture,
and word of the therapist should be dissected and studied
closely, and his entire behavior rehearsed and reenacted.

The degree of the therapist's activity is also a subject full of
controversy. It is sometimes advocated that the "blank wall"
or "sounding board" attitude, and silence or minimal activity
on the part of the therapist are the best technical maneuvers,
while others recommend giving advice or talking a great deal.
Sometimes they even consider the advocacy of physical
contact with the patient.

In my opinion, the therapist's attitude has to do with two
most important aspects: being idiosyncratic and spontaneous.
Insofar as these attitudes are concerned, one may spell out
certain technical guidelines or general principles which should
be kept in mind but not viewed as unconditional authoritative
rules for the therapist to follow. Within the context of these

dimensions the therapist and the patient come face to face. What one should remember is that the patient needs the therapist's objective and novel approach to his problems, while the therapist needs the information which only the patient can provide, thus enabling the therapist, in turn, to reach a specific psychodynamic formulation of the emotional difficulties involved and thereby to be able to help the patient solve these problems.

There are certain essentials for becoming a short-term anxiety-provoking psychotherapist. The knowledge of the theoretical considerations involved in the selection criteria of patients, the technical requirements, the aims and goals, the results obtained, and the experience gained by treating several patients under individual supervision is an obvious prerequisite. Above and beyond these considerations, however, there are certain personality traits which, in my opinion, every psychotherapist must possess. Imagination, flexibility, and a dissatisfaction with the mere narrow gathering of facts are excellent qualities, because they denote inquisitiveness and the curiosity to pursue and understand the patient's problems. In addition, the detached and objective ability to assess the patient's difficulties must be counterbalanced by the intuitive, sympathetic interest in another suffering human being.

The therapist should decide as soon as possible what kind of psychotherapy he plans to employ and, tempting as it may be, he must not rely on the referring source for this decision. The well-known tendency of a beginning and anxious psychotherapist to rely on the superior knowledge of the experienced older referring psychiatrist or on the opinions expressed in the psychiatry record, and the failure to decide for himself as to whether to treat the patient (who may occasionally not be a good candidate for psychotherapy), has led to many a therapeutic tragedy. If he decides to use anxiety-provoking psychotherapy, there are certain tasks which he must do as soon as possible. He must again go all over the whole evaluation process as it was described in the previous chapter. The history-taking of the patient's emotional development should be utilized for the formulation of his psychodynamic hypothesis, and, at the same time, the selection criteria should be reassessed, so that the therapist is satisfied that the patient is indeed a good candidate for this kind of treatment. The preparation of the patient for short-term anxiety-provoking psychotherapy is just as important as the therapist's conviction that he should use this technique. After this, the therapist must, first of all, spend some time in educating the patient regarding what he is to expect. This process is part of the overall structuring of the psychotherapeutic process. McGuire,[1] who has utilized Bruner's[2] original concept, emphasizes that structuring and sequencing play an important role in this kind of treatment, not only during each psychotherapeutic hour but also throughout the entire treatment process itself.

Preparation of the Patient

The patient meets his therapist with certain expectations which have developed as a result of the process of evaluation. Although at first he might not have been as clearly aware of the nature of his emotional problem, as a result of the evaluation interviews he has been able to select one of his various complaints which he wants to eliminate and to assign to it top priority for treatment. Consequently, he expects to be able, more or less, to understand himself and overcome this specific difficulty, which, despite his efforts in the past, he had been unable to solve alone. In other words, a shift has taken place in the patient's expectations — from a wish for symptomatic relief to a wish for a more basic change in attitudes and understanding.

Requirements

The interviews are face-to-face, once a week, forty-five minutes long, and at a specific time. It should be explained to the patient that if he arrives late he cannot expect that the time lost will be made up at the end of the hour, because this will interfere with the timing of the interview of the next patient. If something of importance to the patient is brought up at the end of the hour it should be made clear that it cannot be discussed until the next interview.

The time set aside specifically for the patient may not be utilized by anybody else; therefore, the patient must understand that he will be charged for missed interviews unless the prospective cancellation is discussed with the therapist in advance and an agreement regarding the time is reached between them. It is possible that one may view these requirements as too rigid or artificial. I think that this clear-cut elucidation of the position of the therapist is part and parcel of the education of the patient concerning the psychotherapeutic rules. It shows the patient that the therapist takes his role seriously. An example follows.

A thirty-two-year-old male patient who had difficulties with his girl friends and was worried about the situation following the first two interviews, arrived fifteen minutes late for his third appointment. This was discussed during the interview. He missed the fourth appointment but called up to say that he would be unable to keep it. He did not appear for the fifth appointment and did not telephone.

At this point the therapist wrote him a letter, stating that he was planning to terminate the therapy unless he heard from the patient within a week. The patient called up to say that he was going to keep his next appointment. He arrived early, apologized for the previous cancellations, and started to give some details about how he had forgotten the hour. The therapist interrupted him, stating that it was not a matter of an apology but was something else which, to him, was of much greater importance. He went on as follows: "I take psychotherapy seriously and I assume that my patient also has the same attitude. The kinds of difficulty which you have with women and which we decided to look into and try to disentangle seem to indicate a serious problem which interferes with your whole life, as you yourself have acknowledged. The problem cannot be eliminated unless you are here, for us to understand it and to try to solve it together. Your absence demonstrated to me that your initial interest in this task is dwindling."

The patient was taken aback by this straightforward presentation.

Patient: I did not realize that you are so keenly interested in helping me with my problems. Maybe I was trying to test you?

Doctor: Maybe you were, and this is of importance; but I wonder what you think of all the angry feelings that you expressed at your mother, which took you by surprise after we talked about in the interview. You may remember that you were fifteen minutes late the next time, and after we discussed this delay, I again asked you about your relation to your mother — particularly after your father divorced her. You changed the subject repeatedly from then on, and I brought you back to it over and over. Do you remember?

Patient: Well, yes. I do.

Doctor: How much does your tendency to avoid talking about the subject of your relation with your mother have to do with your missing the subsequent two hours?

The patient was noncommittal. The next hour he recounted a dream about his mother and himself which had bothered him. He said that he had not expected psychotherapy to be so disturbing. He had dealt with his anxiety by evading it — a familiar pattern which he had used in the past.

In reviewing this case in retrospect, it became clear that the therapist's confrontation about the missed appointments seemed to have played a crucial role in stimulating the patient's motivation to continue his treatment, which proceeded fairly uneventfully from then on.

The patient is free to use his hour in any way he sees fit. He may smoke if he so desires. The therapist usually takes notes, although there is some difference of opinion on this point. I, personally, take notes, and I find that it does not interfere with the spontaneity of the communication with the patient. Notes become invaluable to the therapist whenever he wishes to review the trend of a psychotherapeutic process. For example, they help him remember the details and associations of a specific event, or special fantasies which were brought up in relation to a certain dream. Nothing can be more impressive to a patient than to repeat to him his own words, to confront him with his own resistance, to clarify the way he handles his own emotional conflict, and to demonstrate to him a specific pattern of his own behavior. Finally, if an interview is to be tape recorded or videotaped, written permission must always be obtained from the patient. These mechanical devices are invaluable for teaching purposes. At this point I shall summarize the main technical factors of short-term anxiety-provoking psychotherapy which will be discussed in greater detail later on in this chapter.[3]

Role of the Therapist

The therapist encourages the establishment of rapport and tries to create early a therapeutic alliance. He must set up a tentative psychodynamic hypothesis in order to arrive at a formulation of the patient's emotional conflicts, based on the evidence which he has collected during the history-taking, which will guide him throughout the psychotherapeutic process. The therapist tries to investigate and arrive at an agreement with the patient as to what symptoms or inter-personal difficulties, or both, are considered to be of top priority and must be resolved. Furthermore, he must establish how these characteristics are associated with underlying emotional conflicts. This task is referred to as the definition of the patient's emotional problem which must be solved by both the therapist and the patient during the course of the psychotherapy. It is possible that this problem may differ from that which was decided upon during the evaluation. It should be remembered, however, that since the therapist is the one who will treat the patient, his assessment of the problem and his agreement with the patient become the basis for this mutual work.

He may try to convince the patient to modify the problem which is to be solved and to focus upon a new area of emotional conflict, if this becomes necessary as a result of new material which is brought up during the psychotherapy. His specific goal is to concentrate on a circumscribed area of the unresolved emotional conflicts which may be underlying the patient's problem and to teach the patient to become aware of them and to gain objectivity concerning them. He utilizes the patient's positive transference feelings explicitly and early, as the main psychotherapeutic tool. He uses confrontation and clarification in an effort to stimulate the patient to work through the material. In the example of the patient who started to come late and missed his two subsequent appointments, confrontation was used to stimulate the patient's motivation to pursue his treatment. Confrontation is also used to help the patient experience his transference feelings during the interview. The best way to achieve this is by utilizing anxiety-provoking questions.

Clarification is less painful. The therapist, having gathered all the important available facts about a given pattern of the patient's behavior, proceeds systematically to analyze and to assemble all its aspects in detail -- as if putting together the pieces of a jigsaw puzzle — until it appears that the patient has seen the overall picture, understood its purpose, and has experienced the emotions associated with it. From then on, this type of analytic-synthetic method becomes a pattern to be utilized in other situations. The therapist can refer back to this first experience and use it as an example in future sessions. He bypasses character traits consistently, such as masochism, excessive passivity, and dependence, which give rise to therapeutic complications. He prepares the patient to rehearse his reactions and utilize whatever problem-solving techniques he has learned during psychotherapy, so that he may use them effectively to avoid difficulties in the future, after therapy has terminated.

He expects to help the patient achieve a basic change, so far as his interpersonal relationships are involved, as a result of his learning to solve new problems rather than to be satisfied with only symotomatic relief. Finally, he ends the treatment early. These technical points will now be discussed in greater detail under the following headings, which represent the five major phases of short-term anxiety-provoking psychotherapy: (1) The Patient-Therapist Encounter, (2) The Early Treatment, (3) The Height of the Treatment, (4) Evidence of Change, and (5) The Process of Termination.

The Patient-Therapist Encounter

It has long been argued that it is difficult to differentiate clearly between psychiatric evaluation and therapy. Although psychotherapy starts immediately at the first encounter between the patient and his therapist, the therapist must complete the evaluation of the patient's problem as soon as possible. He must do this in order to prepare for the smooth development of the second phase of the treatment, by taking into consideration the patient's expectations about results of the therapy. Thus, he must establish rapport by utilizing the patient's positive feelings, which are usually present at this time. This enables him to set up a therapeutic alliance between the patient and the therapist and to create an atmosphere where learning can take place.

There is a second technical point which has to do with what has already been discussed — namely, the need to have a tentative psychodynamic hypothesis in order to set up a formulation of the patient's emotional problem. The importance of having such a hypothesis cannot be overemphasized, because it is a prerequisite for obtaining a complete history of the patient's emotional development, with special emphasis placed on the interpersonal relations, which give a clear picture of how the patient deals with the realities of the outside world. All this information helps the therapist obtain the evidence necessary for setting up a psychodynamic formulation of the patient's psychopathology, which will act as a guide to him throughout the course of psychotherapy. This is a difficult task. Details of information obtained as a result of persistent questioning are gathered in the therapist's mind and become the pieces of a three-dimensional puzzle which slowly fall in place at different time levels. A picture starts to emerge on one plane which is connected sooner or later by another picture on a different level. The complicated three-dimensional patterns start to merge and help build the skeleton of the psychodynamic edifice which helps in understanding the patient's emotional problem. What is left to be done during the psychotherapy for both the patient and the therapist is to clarify certain areas and consolidate others until the final structure which emerges is firmly established.

The Patient's Expectations

Although certain attempts have been made during the extensive evaluation to assess the patient's expectation of what he hopes to achieve during the psychotherapy, it is important that this be done once more. What are the patient's goals? What does he anticipate will happen during his treatment? What does he expect will be the role of the therapist? What does he want to achieve as a result of therapy? What does he view as his own role during this experience? Some of these questions must be clarified. The first encounter gives the therapist an idea as to what to expect and, in any case, it sets the tone for things to come.

The patient's feelings of enthusiastic anticipation about his treatment, or his disappointment after he has met the therapist, may be significant. Initial transference feelings may be associated and aroused in the patient which could color and influence the rest of the therapy. Thus, the patient's opening remarks and his choice of subject may give a significant clue as to what is to follow. They usually are representative of the patient's style. They are his opening gambit.

A twenty-seven-year-old student who had difficulties with his employer at work started his first interview by giving an elaborate account of his sexual life. When, finally, the therapist asked him why he was going into so many details, the patient looked surprised, and said, "Isn't sex what you psychiatrists are interested in?" The need to please the therapist was an example of his automatic response to people in authority — the very characteristic he resented. When the therapist mentioned that the psychotherapy was not set up for his own interest but was aimed at understanding and solving the patient's emotional problems, he seemed pleased, and said, "Well, maybe, after all, this treatment is going to do me some good!"

Evaluation and History-Taking

It is usually preferable to let the patient open the first interview and talk freely about whatever he wishes; yet, at the same time, tempting as it may be to pursue in greater detail these opening remarks of the patient, this should not alter the therapist's determination to complete the patient's evaluation by obtaining a detailed history. Having emphasized during the first interview that psychotherapy should become a joint venture in which the patient participates actively and not as a passive onlooker, at some appropriate point the therapist should proceed with the history-taking, even if a complete past history has already been obtained during the evaluation interviews. It may seem obvious that everyone knows how to take a history, since this is one of the first techniques that every medical student learns. It is very unfortunate, however, that this is not the case; and, because it has been taken for granted, many a psychiatry resident completes his training and still does not know how to take an adequate psychiatric history.

There are two schools of thought about history-taking. The famous "brown" or "red" history-taking guide book, on which every second-year medical student relies for information concerning what questions to ask during the "system review" or what points not to overlook as he attempts to get the social history, is viewed by him as an instrument which will help him solve the riddle of the patient's diagnosis. He tends to depend heavily upon it in an understandable effort to hide his inexperience. Although it is meant to be only a flexible guideline for the student to use judiciously, most often it is followed rigidly with the result that the history becomes complete, but artificial.

Employing a set of instructions, which offer the patient a list of forced-choice questions which he must answer by a "yes" or "no," is not the best way to take a history. It does not follow, however, that an open-ended question approach is necessarily much better. Although the student may obtain some meaningful information in one area, letting the patient ramble on and on in a guideless way, as often happens, will result in much time being wasted and perhaps some vital clue or bit of information being lost.

It is important, then, that a judicious confrontation by open-ended and forced-choice types of questions, used in such a way as to obtain a clear and continuous picture of the patient's overall emotional development, is the most appropriate way to proceed. Special attention should be focused on the developmental history as well as on interpersonal relationships, particularly with parents, that prevailed during the first few years of life, on the early family atmosphere, on the school history, and on problems that arose during puberty and adolescence. Such information will probably give some clue as to the patient's ability to deal with difficult situations during his adult life in such important areas as his relations with others, his work, and his marriage. The manner in which the patient handles his anxiety should also be surveyed from his earliest years up to the present.

Slowly the areas of conflict and the maladaptive reactions employed to handle them will appear, and the repetitive difficulties in coping with certain hazardous situations will soon start to emerge. At such a point the therapist must ask specific questions; and, from the patient's replies, he must obtain the evidence, to his own satisfaction, as to whether his suspicions about a specific area of emotional difficulty can be confirmed. Sooner or later this will lead, in most cases, to a fairly clear picture of the patient's psychodynamics. A hypothesis, then, based on definite evidence emanating from the patient and not on idle speculation is formulated in the therapist's mind. Up to this time the therapist has used the patient as a source of information; now he needs to obtain from him a systematic statement about what he considers to be the problem he wants to solve during his treatment.

If both the therapist and the patient see eye to eye on this issue, no problem is anticipated. Most of the time, however, this is not the situation; and the patient, as has already been mentioned, must be asked to assign top priority to the area of the emotional problem he wants to solve. The therapist, if he disagrees, must present to the patient what, in his opinion, appears to be a more serious problem. Usually these two positions are not as opposed to each other as they may appear at first glance. What is needed is the establishment of a connection between the underlying conflicts and the super-ficial complaints. This is the task of the therapist. He must try to demonstrate to the patient convincingly and, as completely as it is possible to do, why he disagrees with him. Usually a compromise can be reached, as the following example shows.

A young man who complained of pain in his chest was referred from the medical clinic after having had extensive diagnostic studies, which were negative. He said he was afraid his trouble might be due to some serious disease; he felt sorry for himself. He mentioned, also, that he had difficulty in getting along with men, but he felt equally ill at ease with women. The therapist disagreed with the recommendation of the evaluation team, which had suggested focusing during the treatment on his relations to men. He was of the impression instead that the fear of illness was used as a way of getting sympathy and attention, and also as a way to evade his anger for women, which he feared but was unable to express well. From the history-taking it became clear that the patient as a little boy had obtained sympathy from his "cold" doctor-father only when he was sick. To the therapist his reaction to his mother's rejection seemed to be a bigger problem, and he suggested to the patient that he think about it and be prepared to discuss it during the next hour.

The patient returned after one week, saying that he had given the matter much thought and added that, although the pains in his chest still continued and worried him, he realized that his angry feelings toward women bothered him and he was willing to explore them also. He went on as follows: "My girl friend is very unsympathetic about my pain. She claims that it is all in my mind. This attitude of hers irritates me, as it has always done. At such times I feel sorry for myself and go and talk to the guys in the office. You know, once you talk about illness, such as the flu or something like that, everybody gets interested and has something to say. 'Take aspirin.' 'Don't.' 'Excedrin is better.' 'No. I find a hot bath and a drink works best.' Well, you know all this, but such talk makes me feel better. Mind you, they are not interested in *you*, they are interested in your headache or your cough or in the chest pain. I am not saying that the pain is in my head. It is not. I feel it right here." He pointed to his chest.

The therapist said that he did not doubt in the slightest that the patient had a pain; but what he emphasized was that he could help the patient understand his reactions to this pain which seemed to create problems for him; and he added that, since the x-rays and other findings were negative, this indicated that there was no serious disease present. "After all, muscle spasm can cause pain," he said. "What seems to be the basic problem, in my opinion, is your anger at your mother or at your girl friend. Your fear that the pain is caused by something serious and also your efforts to use this fear in such a way as to get attention when you feel you need it seems to be a secondary reaction. The patient was hesitant but agreed to look into his particular difficulties with women. He went on. "There is something inside me that says, 'Don't do it,' he said, "so I figure that it must be important and that I resist it. I am willing to give it a trial."

Thus, by the end of the first few interviews, the patient's emotional difficulty would have been defined and it was agreed upon that it was the basic emotional problem to be solved during the psychotherapy. Following is another example.

A nineteen-year-old high school senior came to the clinic complaining of being bored and depressed after the death of his mother two years before and of his having difficulty in deciding whether to go to college or join the army. It was thought during the evaluation that an unresolved grief reaction seemed to be the main problem, but the therapist was not exactly sure that this was the only difficulty. In the second interview he was impressed by the fact that this young man had serious difficulties with his father and other male friends, and he pointed this out to the patient. "It seems that your angry outbursts at your friends when they try to advise you about what to do are like your angry outbursts at your father when he inquires about your future career." The patient admitted that he was angry with his father and saw joining the army as a way out of his dilemma. "In Vietnam I could get away from it all." The therapist then asked, "Now, what in your opinion is a bigger problem for you — your feelings of sadness for the loss of your mother or the problem with your father, your friends, and this need to run away." The patient was silent for a while. Finally, he said, "In a way, I know I miss my Mom. She was nice to me and my sadness has a lot to do with the way I feel. But at the present time my big problem is my indecision about the army and college. This is what I want to figure out."

Finally, the therapist must set up certain criteria as to the barest minimum necessary to be achieved during the treatment and make predictions for himself as to whether they can be accomplished.[4] These minimum conditions should be stated in writing, if possible, so that they could be used eventually by those who might be interested in evaluating the results of psychotherapy. Both patient and therapist, as a result of their initial encounter and their different points of view, have a common task, i.e., the solution of the patient's specific emotional problem which must be attempted during the ensuing psychotherapy.

Early Treatment

The Patient

During the early part of the therapy the patient's positive feelings for the therapist are at their height. After having tried repeatedly but unsuccessfully to solve his own difficulties, the patient has reached the point where he sees the possibility of success becoming a reality, and he looks upon the therapist as someone with whose assistance he would be able to finally succeed. Expectations of the therapist's magical ability to produce a cure, if they have persisted until now, are beginning to recede rapidly. The elaborate efforts made by the evaluators and by the therapist should dispel and dissipate any unrealistic expectations still remaining. The patient has been treated as an adult. His role as a participant — as someone who has the capabilities of working hard and of solving his own problems, which have been emphasized — gives him a sense of well-being. He is grateful to his therapist. Furthermore, he feels excited as a result of the work on the definition of the emotional problem. A wider horizon is opened to him. Not only may his symptoms improve but he may now have the opportunity to learn more about himself and to effect a change. He is imbued with eager anticipation.

This is how one patient expressed himself: "I never expected that psychotherapy could be like this. Although I knew that there were not going to be any miracles and that it was not like going to see your family doctor, and although everybody made it quite clear that it was up to me to work and solve my problems, I somehow, deep inside, couldn't believe it. The first two sessions made all the difference. It is hard to explain how. I know, realistically, that we decided on what we had to do. This, I am sure, helped a lot. It clarified things. But — what was even more important — I felt convinced that it was really up to me. I felt that you trusted me and had confidence in my being able to do the work. This was very satisfying. After each of the sessions I went to my room and did a lot of thinking. The amazing thing was that I started to think in a different way. This was very exhilarating. The possibility that I might discover a new way of looking at myself made a great difference. I just want to mention this today because it is very important to me." These words give a vivid picture of the early phase of the treatment.

The Therapist

The therapist not only must not ignore such positive attitudes but must take advantage of them and utilize them explicitly and vigorously. Here is the golden opportunity to bring the old family conflicts into the atmosphere of the newly developing doctor-patient relationship. The therapist must then confront the patient with his transference feelings and use them as the main psychotherapeutic tool.

The term "transference" must be defined. It is an emotional interaction between two people, having both conscious and unconscious aspects.[5] Freud's[6] discovery of transference became the basis of psychoanalysis, as well as of all kinds of psychodynamic psychotherapy. Freud himself thought, however, that transference occurred not only during but also outside of psychoanalysis, and Glover[7] considered it as "a normal affective phenomenon governed by unconscious mechanisms of displacement and promoting social adaptation." In this way transference is not considered as applying not only to neurotic patients but to everyone, including the therapist. In addition to Freud and Glover, several psychoanalysts have been interested in transference phenomena and have written extensively about it. Recently, Greenson[8] emphasized that repetition and inappropriateness are outstanding characteristics of transference, and Alexander and French[9] stressed that a distinction should be made between transference reactions adequate to realistic present situations and significant repetitive reactions to a person from the past.

An example of an instantaneous development of transference that relates to past experiences is found in a patient of mine in her third year of psychoanalysis who admitted with some embarrassment that she was surprised to find out that my nose was "perfectly normal." When I asked her to elaborate, she admitted that ever since her first evaluation interview she had felt sorry for me because of my "crooked nose." This conviction of hers was associated with her wish to make men turn into women, which had been worked through very slowly during her psychoanalytic treatment, before her final willingness to give up this neurotic idea. It was at this point that she was willing to acknowledge to herself that her analyst's nose (which was supposed to have been "flattened out and eaten by disease") was "perfectly normal."

The emphasis up to now has been on the patient's positive feelings. This, of course, does not mean that ambivalent feelings do not exist. It simply means that the positive ones predominate. This obvious distinction should also be kept in mind because feelings from the past should be differentiated from those of the present. Thus, the patient's anger at the therapist may be perfectly legitimate, justifiable, appropriate, and realistic, and may have nothing to do with past situations.

A further distinction is also necessary at this point: one should differentiate clearly between transference and transference neurosis. Transference neurosis is the transfer of all conscious and unconscious fantasies, emotions, and attitudes for all people in the past on to the therapist during the height of the psychoanalysis of neurotic patients. Glover states: "Everything that takes place during the analytic session, every thought, action, gesture, with reference to the external thought and action, every inhibition or thought or action relates to the transference situation between the patient and his analyst." Although the line of demarcation between these two terms may not be clear cut, it is helpful to keep them apart. For practical purposes, it is in degree that they differ.

In any case, the therapist must take advantage of the long time lag in the appearance of the transference neurosis in fairly healthy patients. The longer this time lag, the healthier the patient. The analyst, by use of free association, has access to the patient's fantasies and unconscious conflicts and is therefore able to analyze the transference neurosis successfully before psychoanalysis ends. The transference neurosis is, of course, an intense experience. In one form or another, however, and after some time has passed, the transference neurosis will appear during the course of psychotherapy. If the therapist lets this happen, invariably complications are likely to develop which may prove to be insoluble, because the therapist is limited by the once-a-week, face-to-face interactions and has at his disposal only limited access to the patient's unconscious conflicts. He is, therefore, unable to analyze successfully the transference neurosis, and the therapy ends in an impasse. This is one of the main reasons why the therapy must be conducted with relative speed and must end quickly.

From all this it should be clear that the therapist should be on the alert to pick up the early manifestations or delays in the appearance of the patient's transference feelings for him. Thus, as soon as the patient makes reference to him, even in a casual way, the therapist must express interest and be willing to discuss it, even if this happens in the first or second interview. The therapist does not have to wait until transference appears as a resistance. This principle, which has been recommended by Freud and several analysts, involves the unrealistic and unconscious aspects of the transference feelings which should not be gratified or manipulated. On the contrary, what is emphasized in short-term anxiety-provoking psychotherapy is that confrontation of the positive transference does not need to be be postponed. The patient is capable of examining every aspect of his behavior, tracing the origins of his emotional problem in the past, and seeing for himself the ways in which his conflicting desires give rise to symptoms that have produced his difficulties. To do all this, he must first understand his reactions toward his therapist. The therapist, in turn, must use his wisdom in reference to this which, in my opinion, is what Felix Deutsch[10] calls "the correct use of the doctor-patient relationship." In a different dimension, this is an ingredient in the education of the patient concerning psychotherapy, because it involves the teaching of the rules — an integral part of the preparation for the work to be done during the height of the treatment.

The Height of the Treatment

The following case is an example of a patient at the height of therapy.

A thirty-two-year-old man, while on his honeymoon, suddenly developed acute obsessive-compulsive symptoms consisting of a need to pick up papers or pieces of metal from the floor or from the street. He had the urge to make sure he had picked up everything and to know that every-thing was clean. He was also tormented by the preoccupying thought that he might have been in some way responsible for his father's death, although he realized the absurdity of such thoughts. He was intelligent, he related very well, and had a good work history and fairly good relations with other people. He responded well during the evaluation interview and was eager for help because his symptoms interfered with his marriage and his work.

His father had died six months before the treatment was started. He said that although he cried during his father's funeral, he had noticed on other similar occasions an inappropriate tendency to laugh. Soon after his father's death he met a young woman, fell in love with her, and, after a courtship of four months which involved satisfactory sexual relations, they decided to be married. While on their honeymoon, his wife received a wedding present. She hurriedly opened the package, and, in her delight at its contents, she forgot to gather up the wrappings that were strewn all over the floor of the hotel room. When the patient saw them he meticulously started to pick them up and experienced a feeling of intense anger as he did so.

He always came early for his interviews, related well to his therapist, and made a genuine effort to understand himself. At the fourth inter-view, he arrived ten minutes late and was silent when the therapist pointed this out. After a moment, he turned to him angrily and said, "You're blaming me for being late." The therapist emphasized that this was not his intention, at which the patient apologized, was silent for a while, and then said that an entirely irrelevant episode from his child-hood had crossed his mind. He was encouraged to talk about it, and, as he reminisced, he said that when he was twelve years old he liked to go fishing with his father. On one occasion he dropped his fishing rod accidentally, and, as he tried to retrieve it he almost overturned the boat. His father was very angry at him, and said, "You are always so careful. How can you be so careless now? I could have drowned!" He said he remembered being angry at that time and that this irrelevant thought had entered his mind: "How can my dad be so sloppy and leave his desk in such a mess"! He again became silent. When asked what he was thinking, he said he had noticed several sheets of paper lying on the psychiatrist's desk. Upon being asked what this reminded him of, he answered, "Dad did not give up. He called me to his study and kept on lecturing to me about safety. I didn't care. The only thing I could think about was the sheets of paper strewn all over his desk," and then, with a smile, he added, "You have a cute secretary."

At the next interview the patient was fifteen minutes late. He said that his compulsive symptom had been very bothersome for the whole week. He then announced that he had an irrelevant urge to take the wastepaper basket and strew its contents all over the doctor's desk. At this point he became visibly anxious, his hands started to shake, and he said that this thought was in some way connected with the fear that he was somehow responsible for his father's death. As the therapist drew a parallel between his attitude toward him and his attitude toward his father, the patient admitted having the fantasy that he wished the therapist would drop dead suddenly. "Then I can sleep with your secretary," he added. The patient was on time for the next appointment and told about the following dream: He had gone hunting with a girl friend when, suddenly, a huge ostrich appeared and started to chase him. Although he wanted to kill the bird to impress his girl friend, he was unable to do so because his gun "would not fire." He woke up feeling somewhat relieved. When asked about his association to the dream, he remembered that when he was six years old he tried to peek at his older sister while she was taking a shower and felt vaguely that this was a wrong thing to do. Later on during the interview he remembered his father returning from fishing. He had caught several fish, and they were all lying on the kitchen table. What had impressed him most was a rainbow trout that appeared to have been decapitated accidentally. He shuddered at the idea and was visibly shaken. In the next few interviews he talked a great deal about the relations he had had with women. He had loved to give parties, and women were very much attracted to him, but he had had a tendency to disregard his own date and flirt with his best friend's girl. He said that his mother always liked to give dinner parties when his father was on fishing trips. His father disapproved of this. For those dinner parties, he remembered, his sister always dressed seductively. He remembered having dreams of being married to his sister but always woke up feeling very anxious because a dark figure would invariably threaten him. He also noted that his wife looked very much like his sister.

The psychodynamics of this case are obvious. The therapist brought together repeatedly the attitude of the patient toward his father and toward the therapist. His anger at the therapist and his wish that he would drop dead were associated with the fishing episode, the decapitated rainbow trout, and his father's death. His attitude toward his sister, his marriage after his father's death, and his wishes for the psychiatrist's secretary were also linked together. As a result of the interviews the patient reexperienced his past emotional conflicts with his father which were underlying his obsessive symptoms and thus he was able to solve his emotional problem. His symptoms improved dramatically and soon disappeared. Therapy was discontinued after the sixteenth interview. Three years later he was asymptomatic.

The Therapist
The height of the treatment is characterized by the repeated efforts of the therapist to concentrate in the areas of unresolved conflicts which underlie the patient's emotional problem and to avoid the difficulties involving character traits which are considered to be more primitive. To accomplish this, the therapist utilizes confrontation and anxiety-provoking questions in order to bring into the open the patient's emotions to help them become "alive," so to speak, during the interview in order to help him look into the areas of difficulty he tends to avoid. These techniques stimulate the patient to reexamine past conflicts and instruct him repeatedly how to analyze, scrutinize, and understand his reactions and his emotional behavior. Confrontation is an invaluable technical tool of short-term anxiety-provoking psychotherapy. It is a forceful approach which the therapist chooses to use in order to achieve his therapeutic goals because he is convinced that it will produce better results than a gentler, more persuasive technique. Confrontation creates pain, but the therapist is convinced as a result of the detailed assessment of the patient's strengths of character that he deals with someone who can withstand a considerable degree of strain. Finally, he encourages the patient to employ new ways to deal with his conflicts and to solve his problem. Let us now consider these points in greater detail.

Concentration on areas of unresolved emotional conflicts. The therapist is aided in this task by his psychodynamic hypothesis of the patient's difficulties. He then proceeds to get more information from the patient about past experiences and to assess his evidence. Sooner or later the transference may appear as a resistance, and at this point the therapist switches from getting information about conflicting situations with people in the past to confronting the patient with his resistant feelings toward the therapist in the present. As soon as this has been accomplished the therapist may resume getting information about past events.

One could conceptualize the work of the therapist as a walk on two parallel tracks. He steps at first on one and then, after a while, he shifts to the other. One track deals with the transference relationship; the other is concerned with the patient's past. As long as the patient is able to stay on the subject which is being worked through currently in the treatment, there is no need for the therapist to bring the transference into the open. Sooner or later, however, resistances start to appear. The whole tone of the interviews start to change. Instead of the smooth narrative and eager attempts of the patient to understand what happened, silences interrupted by efforts to avoid and to change the subject start to appear. The patient may even hint at the transference by shifting and talking in oblique ways about the therapist. The whole interview seems fragmented. At such time the therapist should shift his attention to difficulties arising within the transference relationship, which must be clarified before the therapy can proceed smoothly again.

In addition to confrontation, clarification is also an important technical tool. Whenever he has a clarification to make, the therapist uses (as already mentioned) clear-cut examples which have come up within the context of the transference relationship, and, at such times, he may quote verbatim the patient's statements from past interviews. This usually makes a very marked impression on the patient, who may be startled, surprised, or even shocked to hear his own words spoken back to him. It is like hearing one's own voice on a tape recorder. There is usually a sense of slight embarrassment on the part of many of us on such occasions. "Do I really sound like that?" we ask. This is due, possibly, to our inability to see or hear ourselves from the outside or to conceptualize the way we really look or sound to other people. In this sense, note-taking comes in handy for the therapist, because if he does decide later to quote the patient he must do so correctly.

Slowly the conflicts start to emerge, as well as the emotions and the reactions utilized to handle them. Following is an example.

A twenty-year-old student, who was treated for a depression, had talked repeatedly about his tendency to look down on himself, not to care about his appearance, and generally to let himself drift. He had said in several interviews that when he was young he got a lot of attention from both of his parents (who were obsessed about cleanliness) when he dirtied his clothes while playing. He had, in passing, during the first interview, admitted that he, as a child, purposely smeared mud on his shirt. He also had mentioned having begged for money once from an old woman while playing in the park. She, seeing that he was well-dressed but covered with mud, felt sorry for him, gave him a quarter, and washed off his coat for him herself.

In his interview the patient told how he had spent all of his money and had gone out of his way to ask several of his friends for loans. He also complained of feeling weak, incapable of doing anything well, and of being "deflated" and sad. After hearing all this for a while, the doctor exclaimed, "You emphasize how sad you are, but we know you enjoy the attention you get from being broke, from begging, and from being helpless." "Good point," the patient said, and was silent for a while. He then added, "I understand, but you don't seem to care how I feel"; and then much more emphatically he went on, "You are so disinterested you don't give a damn. You don't give me a thing in the way of help."

Doctor: Like what, for example?

Patient: Food for thought, anything, any old crumb.

Doctor: So. Although you profess to understand, you are, right this minute, still begging, asking me to give, begging for crumbs.

Patient (pause): Damn you!

Doctor: I can see you are angry when your manipulations fail. The question is whether begging for money and for bread crumbs of "smearing your clothes with mud" is to your best interest. Yet we do know that you are capable at other times of getting along without all this self pity.

Patient: I know what you mean. I am surprised, however, that you do know all this.

Doctor: At this time you may interpret what I told you as having given you those bread crumbs. Actually I gave you back what *you told me* in our first interview.

Patient: I had completely forgotten! (He looked thoroughly surprised.)

114

This type of clarification of the patient's behavior was used several times during the psychotherapy, until the patient seemed to refer to "his sad sack ways" with amusement.

Active avoidance of characterological complications. Knight[11] emphasizes the importance of "the optimal level of positive feeling in the patient which is conducive for effective psychotherapeutic work," and Alexander stresses that if the transference neurosis is "allowed to reach great intensity" it can "impair the therapy." These technical points, discussed already, are best achieved, in my opinion, only if the therapist actively avoids dealing with deep-seated characterological traits in the patient, such as excessive passivity, narcissistic gratification, or dependence. When the patient introduces such material, it is best for the therapist to intervene and change the subject, despite the fact that this may tend to make the patient angry.

A thirty-two-year-old single obese male teacher had a quarrel with a colleague. The episode reminded him of a similar experience when he was in college and his roommate had succeeded in taking his girl friend away from him. He said that at that time he was so angry he felt hungry and had gone to the most high-priced restaurant and "spent a fortune" eating the most expensive foods. From then on, he continued to talk about his enormous enjoyment of eating and of food, as he had done in previous interviews. This was his favorite reaction to competitive and frustrating situations. The therapist cut short these ruminations by asking for details about the recent encounter with the other teacher.

Use of anxiety-provoking questions. The fact that the patient must become aware of his feelings "alive," so to speak, during the interview, has been emphasized already. This can best be done by bringing to the patient's attention the negative feelings he experiences toward his therapist because of the use of anxiety-provoking questions. This initiates the final stage of this phase of short-term psychotherapy, when the patient must be confronted with his anger, fear, anxiety, and sadness, which result from the examination of the areas of emotional conflict that underlie his problem. It is understandable, of course, that the patient has evaded, more or less, such painful feelings. Now it is time that they should be brought into the open more systematically and understood more clearly. The patient, by expressing these unpleasant emotions toward his therapist without being judged, experiences what Alexander calls "a corrective emotional experience" with all its therapeutic value.

The therapist, as a result of his previous work on the patient's positive transference, has established himself as an ally, a trustworthy teacher, and a reliable friend. Thus, he is now able to increase the patient's desire to understand his conflicts, even at the expense of some pain.

Keeping the patient's energy within the problem area, as emphasized by Semrad,[12] is a crucial technical procedure in short-term psychotherapy, but this is no easy task.

In another interview, a patient I have already mentioned, who complained of chest pain and talked at length about feeling sorry for himself and about his need to be taken care of, was recounting with much emotion how he managed to get his friends to reassure him. He went on, "They know I'm miserable, that I don't have much stamina, that I am so strong — I mean, so weak." The therapist thought it was appropriate to utilize this slip of the tongue, to show the patient how he used weakness to cover up his strength. "Are you strong?" the therapist asked. The patient blushed. Looking annoyed, he denied it vehemently and emphasized that he did not "believe in all this Freud stuff." But the therapist persisted. He went back relentlessly to the conflict, despite the patient's annoyance, and gave him specific examples. The patient finally retorted, "You keep on needling me and it hurts, but you may be right. I shall think about it."

The therapist's counter-transference feelings also play an important role. He must be aware of this so that he does not use anxiety-provoking questions to punish the patient, to see the patient suffer, or to enjoy a position of superiority. It is clear that such attitudes will create difficulties, and it is because of this that the therapist should have had psychotherapy or a personal analysis as a part of his education, so as to be at least partially aware of any of his sadistic tendencies.

This type of persistent work and anxiety-provoking questioning is difficult for residents to learn to employ, and it is particularly important that the supervisor help them to become aware of their own feelings and reactions. One of our residents was repeatedly unable to deal with his counter-transference feelings for a seductive female patient who was in the process of expressing (in a roundabout way at first, but progressively more openly) her positive transference feelings for him. For example, when she talked about her sexual involvement with men who had the physical characteristics of her therapist, he ignored her remarks and changed the subject repeatedly. She soon became angry and started to criticize him at an increasing rate. The case was being pre-sented to a group of residents as a teaching exercise, and this made the task more difficult for the therapist. Tension was rising, and it was obvious that, unless the issue was dealt with directly, the therapy would be unsuccessful. At this point, the resident was encouraged to tackle the transference issue head on. After three agonizing interviews, the therapist, urged and supported by the group, was able (to his own amazement) to deal with the transference, counter-transference issues. The ensuing relief on the part of the patient was just as great as the general enthusiasm which his interpretation produced on both his colleagues and his supervisor.

The therapist demonstrates repeatedly the pattern the patient has employed in order to deal with his conflicts. Again and again he uses, and quotes from, the patient's interview material and from the transference relationship notes. He urges the patient to look at the pattern of his behavior and helps him to learn how his present-day interpersonal relation-ships are associated with his past neurotic difficulties, and how, for example, his regressive behavior or his tendency to act in a certain way in order to avoid his unpleasant feelings have created unnecessary complications in his life and caused him much discomfort. By concentrating and focusing on the understanding of the means he has used to avoid anxiety, the therapist helps the patient to examine, and repeatedly re-examine, past problems in the light of the present situations, and to experiment with new ways to solve his emotional problem. His role, thus, is clearly one of an unemotionally involved teacher.

117

The Patient

The patient, as we have seen, is becoming aware of his feelings, positive and negative, during the interview. He soon starts to raise questions on his own and tries to find the answers to them without needing to rely exclusively on his therapist's probing. As a result of his own self-questioning and the persistent and relentless anxiety-provoking work of the therapist, the patient slowly allows himself to experience painful reactions, and his motivation to come to grips with and solve his emotional problem becomes intensified. When he starts, during his treatment, to ask the kinds of questions about himself which might have been raised by the therapist, this is a sign that the psychotherapy is proceeding well.

One evidence that the patient is learning to solve emotional problems is his ability to bring into his interviews spontaneous associations which reenforce or add to the understanding of the emotional difficulties discussed during the previous interview, as if there had been no interruption of one week. The patient gradually becomes convinced that he must face up to his painful affects and interpersonal difficulties.

At some point, the patient usually identifies with the therapist.[13] The distinction should be made here between imitation and identification. The former involves paying lip service to, or agreeing with, the therapist's words without understanding what they mean. Identification, on the other hand, is a dimension of the learning process which involves motivation and selectivity and which encourages independence. It gives the patient an opportunity to make free choices. Interference with identification may become a hindrance to learning and may develop into the crucial point of failure in the psychotherapeutic process.

As the patient's curiosity rises, his motivation increases. Instead of avoiding and evading his painful feelings, he now knows that he must bring them into the open and examine the underlying conflicts that give rise to them. When the emotional problem is finally solved, the patient experiences a profound sense of satisfaction. On the cognitive level, this feeling is similar to what one experiences when he masters a difficult situation or solves a complicated mathematical problem. Furthermore, the realization that he was able to master his tangled interpersonal difficulties with their all-powerful emotions — something he has been unable to do before — gives him a feeling of liberation and his self-esteem is augmented. Relaxation of the probing on the part of the therapist reenforces the patient's reward and not only contributes to a decrease in tension but also gives rise to a sense of well-being.

Evidence of Change

The Therapist

When the therapist is able to demonstrate repeatedly, and to the patient's satisfaction, that the emotional conflicts, as seen in the transference relationship, are a repetition of the patient's interpersonal relationships with people in the past and to show how such difficulties have been handled in the past, how they have created his current entanglements, and how the patient has learned new ways to deal with them and is able to solve them, a great deal has been accomplished. But he must not rest upon his laurels. He must first look for evidence that this has really happened. Hints that it is occurring may emerge as a result of a certain reduction of tension which he notices is taking place during the psycho-therapeutic interviews. Tangible demonstration of progress in the patient's behavior must now be shown to occur outside the interview periods.

Sooner or later the patient gives signs that improvement in interpersonal relationships, in areas where difficulties previously occurred, is taking place. Such tangible evidence of progress should alert the therapist to the realization that termination should be considered. The possibility that a flight into health may be taking place must be considered by the therapist. One can easily distinguish, however, between this kind of solid demonstration of improvement, both inside and outside the psychotherapy, and some action taken by the patient to run away from his problem. When the therapist is also able to encourage the patient to utilize finally these newly developed problem-solving capabilities in other areas of emotional conflict in order to use them effectively in the future, he has succeeded in his task.

The Patient

The patient's abilities to give examples to prove that he is utilizing what he has learned during the therapeutic situation are the best evidence that such new learning has taken place as a result of the treatment. This is, I assume, what Alexander means by "interpretative learning," and Freud by "the process of reeducation." The reader should be cautioned here about the use of the word "learning," which usually implies only an intellectual acquisition of information to be used subsequently. The learning that takes place as a result of short-term anxiety-provoking psychotherapy has an emotional component, also, but this should come as no surprise. It should be remembered however that what Strupp[14] calls "therapeutic learning" depends to a large extent on the emotional tie between the patient and his therapist, and is therefore "predominantly experiential." As has already been mentioned, it has been shown that the learning of autonomic responses can take place in animals. Is it possible, then, that emotional learning can take place in humans?

The Process of Termination

The Therapist

Satisfied that meaningful progress has taken place, but realizing that all difficulties have not yet been overcome, the therapist must avoid the temptation of prolonging the treatment. He not only must be modest enough to realize that he is not indispensable to the patient but he must also remember that there are certain behavior patterns which cannot be altered by psychotherapy. The therapist's attitude toward early termination plays a very crucial role at this juncture. His counter-transference may be prejudiced against termination; his narcissism and his own intellectual curiosity may not only interfere with, but also prolong, the treatment unnecessarily. Young residents are sometimes fascinated both by the "material" and also by the desire to become "amateur psychoanalysts." They are inclined, then, to prolong psychotherapy, hoping to turn it into quasi-psychoanalysis. This tendency is also caused by the attitude of those residents' supervisors who, as analysts, have abandoned psychotherapy long ago and have tended to think of it as a second-best alternative compared with psychoanalysis. In their capacity as supervisors of psychiatry residents, they tend to encourage the prolongation of the treatment. There should be a choice not as to what is the "best" treatment but as to what is the "best" treatment for *whom* and for *what.*

At times, a patient who may show early improvement is treated for several years without any further evidence of progress. Actually, he may be worse off for having become dependent upon the therapist. This, in part, may be due to the false impression that improvement can result only after long treatment and that any other kind of success is only short-lived. Glover gives an example of an obsessive patient who improved after being treated for only a few months. In a casual, accidental follow-up thirty years later, the improvement had been maintained with no evidence of any returning symptoms. Fenichel[15] also emphasizes that some patients with obsessive-compulsive symptoms of short duration can improve rapidly. Thus, at times, these early improvements are long-lasting.

The therapist must watch for hints about termination emanating from the patient; or, if they are not forthcoming, he must initiate the talk about termination himself and emphasize that he trusts the patient to carry on his work alone. At this point the therapist concentrates on working through the patient's ambivalent feelings, which usually predominate at times when termination is contemplated. Separation and loss are invariably painful. The therapist must help the patient to recognize that positive and negative emotions may coexist at such times and may be unusually strong. It should be remembered that such emotions are, in reality, aimed at the therapist, although they may have existed at times of separations in the past. Keeping the discussion, then, focused on the present relationship and the prospect of its ending helps to overcome this phase fairly quickly. Otherwise, prolonged discussion of previous separations tends to lengthen the treatment.

After talking about the prospect of termination, a young woman discussed a dream during her next session: She was walking alone on a narrow street when she noticed that her therapist was driving a huge convertible car full of beautiful blondes. She waved at the therapist as he passed by, but he paid no attention to her. Instead, he seemed to laught at a joke made by one of the girls. Then she realized suddenly, to her horror, that the car was on a dead-end street and that it was going to crash. She called out, without being heard. She screamed just before the car hit a brick wall. She rushed to the scene of the crash and by performing mouth-to-mouth resuscitation, she was able to save the therapist's life. By the time she came for her appointment she had analyzed her jealousy, had recognized that the blondes represented other patients who were going to take her place after the end of her treatment. She was disturbed, however, by the thought that she had wished the accident to occur. The therapist explained to her that such emotions were to be expected at a time of separation and that, because they exist, it does not mean that her good responses toward him in the past have disappeared. "After all," he said, "you did save my life with a kiss"!

Part of this work involves making an effort to predict the patient's future course on the basis of what was learned during the treatment and to help to prepare him for his life after psychotherapy has ended. The therapist should encourage the patient to talk about his expectations of what could happen after psychotherapy is concluded. Again, here the role of the therapist has to do with the education of the patient concerning his future. The emphasis should be on encouraging him to take over the role of the therapist as it was formulated during psychotherapy and to make it a part of himself after the treatment is terminated. Thus, the patient should be expected to continue to raise questions about himself which he must try to answer and to anticipate hazardous situations which are likely to produce crises and cause him to become anxious. He should be warned that during such times he *may* revert back to some of his old ways, but he must persist in trying to solve the emotional conflict which is responsible for the crisis in the same way that he has done during his treatment. Teaching the patient to anticipate is a crucial dimension of the termination phase. If this process of reeducation, with its emphasis on preparing the patient for the future, is successful, it carries with it the promise of victory far greater than what was achieved during psychotherapy. Learning a new way of looking at and questioning himself offers the patient the key to overcoming his future emotional difficulties. It is like a vaccine which immunizes him from future ills.

Formal agreement about termination should be reached as soon as possible, but this should be done in a flexible way. We have been unwilling to set up artificial time limits, such as a fixed number of interviews. Every patient should be given time enough to solve his emotional problems, provided he does not take advantage of this to unnecessarily prolong his psychotherapy.

The Patient

When the patient starts to experiment successfully on his own, outside the treatment period, as a result of his solid problem-solving accomplishments during the psychotherapy, he begins to wonder whether termination should be considered. At such times he feels confident that he can face the future with the new weapons he has acquired, and, as already mentioned, he gives hints to the therapist in the form of such questions and comments as: "Where do we go from here"? or "It seems that we have accomplished what we set out to do." He anxiously and eagerly expects his therapist's agreement, even though, at the same time, he feels sad at the prospect of losing the therapist who has been an ally and a friend, and of ending psychotherapy, which has been, on the whole, a meaningful experience for him. Ultimately, the wish to be independent, to trust himself, and to experiment with his new freedom are stronger and healthier desires than the wish to perpetuate the relationship with his therapist.

8

RESULTS

I am aware, of course, that the research design of our various studies requires tightening, that the evidence presented may not be sufficient to permit unequivocal conclusions, and that there are deficiencies in our findings insofar as scientific method is concerned. Nevertheless our findings are significant if they are considered seriously and not dismissed quickly in an effort to discredit psychotherapy, as has often been done. No convincing explanations are intended, rather it is hoped that the reader will draw his own conclusions about the efficacy and value of this kind of psychotherapy.

Our preliminary findings in 1960[1] were, on the basis of twenty-one patients seen in follow-up interviews, from six months to two years after psychotherapy: (1) there was only moderate symptomatic relief; (2) the patients described psychotherapy as a "new learning" experience; (3) there seemed to be a restoration of the patient's self-esteem; (4) the psychotherapy had helped the patients to deal successfully with an emotional crisis which they had previously been unable to conquer; and (5) there was a change from the patient's original expectations of the results of treatment. We were particularly interested in the first two findings. Since for many patients the symptoms had improved only moderately, could the treatment be considered successful? We learned quickly to avoid value judgments, such as good or bad, successful or unsuccessful, cure or non-cure. On close questioning of these patients it was clear that, although in some the symptoms had persisted, their attitude toward the symptoms had changed. They were less bothered by them, or they seemed to have learned to live with them. "The fear of cats is still there somewhere," said a young female student, "but I do not feel compelled to flee as I used to before. They may not be my favorite animal and I doubt that I would have them as my pets, but there they are — they should be reckoned with."

The second finding, namely, that the patients had learned something new, was intriguing. This learning experience was described by them as something "unusual," "new," or as a "unique" experience in their life. These observations stimulated us to pursue our investigation, and we decided to collect verbatim quotations of our patients' statements about the results of short-term psychotherapy and compare their statements with those of other patients in order to obtain as accurate a picture as possible of how they viewed their therapy in retrospect.

Four years later, in 1964, our follow-up observations[2] were essentially the same as in the first ones; however, on closer examination of the patients' statements, improvement in their self-esteem appeared to be the most striking finding. They felt better and seemed to be contented with themselves. This was in sharp contrast with the way they felt about themselves before receiving psychotherapy. These feelings, furthermore, seemed to point to the development of an attitude of contentment about having worked hard in psychotherapy, in essence, about a job well done. Although the patients had positive feelings for their therapists, who were viewed as those who had helped them and who acted as catalysts or as teachers, it was clear that the resulting self-confidence was obviously the reward for the patients' labors and the credit went primarily to the patients themselves. This is how a patient put it: "It is as if I had been reborn. I know it sounds foolish, but this is the only way to approximate the way I feel. The amazing thing about it is that I never knew I had that potential in myself. It was my doctor, with his questions, that helped bring it into the open. For this I am grateful to him. But once it emerged, this previously hidden ability of mine grew larger and stronger. It was I who started asking questions to myself even when I was alone. I know this — that the job was done. I have been looking into myself ever since, and I feel fine. I like myself." This clear expose needs no commentary.

Returning to the question of symptomatic improvement, we were again struck by its partial change. Symptomatic improvement has been looked upon by some investigators as the sole criterion for assessing the results of psychotherapy. In our view, psychodynamic change was of much greater importance, because, as has already been emphasized, psychiatric symptoms are looked upon as end results or postures which the patient is forced to take when he is confronted with an emotional conflict. As Malan put it, "emotional health cannot simply be equated with the absence of symptoms."[3] An example is shown in the following case.

A twenty-two-year-old man had received psychotherapy in another city for two years because of anxiety associated with compulsive stealing. He said that his therapist on two occasions had gone out of his way to write letters for him and protect him when he was faced with serious prospects of being arrested. After a while he was symptom free. He came to our clinic three years later, referred by a judge, because he had been caught stealing. When asked if he wanted psychotherapy, he said that he did not need it but had to accept treatment because, otherwise, he would have to go to jail. Then he went on, "After all, my treatment cured my nervousness. What else is there to be done?" When asked if he was bothered by this tendency to steal, he answered in the negative. He then added, somewhat sheepishly, "The only thing is that I must be careful so as not to be caught the next time."

Although this might be considered as a symptomatic improvement, there is no evidence that he had changed psychodynamically in any way, because he continued to perform his antisocial acts without any understanding of the underlying reasons.

Change in the patient as a result of an intrapsychic alteration, or as a result of rearrangements in the patient's environment, should be clearly differentiated. In our experience, short-term anxiety-provoking psychotherapy produces limited intra-psychic changes. It seems as a result of these changes that the patient is able to deal with environmental pressures in different and more efficient ways for himself. We have made no effort to alter the environment in order to make the patient happy or comfortable, or to help him cover up his problems. This point, it is hoped, has been made clear by now.

Since these preliminary observations were encouraging, we decided to investigate more systematically the results of our treatment. We decided then to have the patient seen by the same evaluator both before and after psychotherapy. As a result of this third study, it was observed that the majority of the patients had developed new adaptive attitudes to deal with their emotional difficulties and attributed this to increased self-esteem and self-understanding. Many patients were able to use what was learned during their treatment in an effort to solve their newest problems. This aspect had not been looked into very carefully in the past, and, in our opinion, it seemed to be the most striking discovery.

We decided, therefore, to set up a controlled study in an effort to assess as systematically as possible what changes could be attributed to short-term anxiety-provoking psychotherapy in patients who were selected according to our original criteria and were treated according to the technical requirements already described, while other patients, selected similarly, had to wait. In this fourth study the patients were designated alternately as "experimental" and "control" and were matched according to sex and age. They were also subdivided into two groups, ranging from seventeen to twenty-one and from twenty-one to forty years of age.

The patients were seen by two independent evaluators both before and after the psychotherapy. The control patients waited while the experimental patients were treated. After the psychotherapy of each experimental patient was finished, the control patient was seen again by the original evaluators, in order to assess what changes had taken place in him during the waiting period. After this, each control patient started his treatment. Again, after the psychotherapy was terminated, the controls were also seen by the original evaluators. Both groups were subsequently followed as long as possible.

The difficulties of such a study are innumerable. By the end of 1967, out of thirty-five experimental and thirty-six control patients, several were lost before, and some after, the end of psychotherapy. In addition, among the control patients, some decided by the end of the waiting period that they did not want therapy. In the final report,[4] the total numbers involved only fourteen experimental and eighteen control patients. By mid-1968 a few more patients had finished therapy, but the numbers are too small for statistical purposes. As one may expect, there are obvious differences between patients who wait and patients who are treated, and our study seems to favor the treated patients over the untreated ones. I suspect, furthermore, that there was bias in favor of obtaining good results in both groups of patients — the majority of whom were students — as well as in the evaluators' estimation of the problem. Despite these shortcomings, as I said previously, these findings are significant.

Classification of Results

The results of short-term anxiety-provoking psychotherapy may be considered under three main categories of change: (1) intrapsychic, (2) interpersonal, and (3) psychodynamic.

1. Intrapsychic changes, as reported by patients
   a. Moderate symptomatic relief
   b. Improvement in self-esteem
   c. Change from the original expectations of the results of psychotherapy
   d. Awareness about psychotherapy had changed and it was described as a "new learning experience"
   e. Old attitudes replaced by new ones, which, in the patients' opinion, were more adaptive ones
   f. Problem-solving developed during psychotherapy
   g. Problem-solving techniques learned during psychotherapy were

    used to solve new problems arising in everyday life after treatment
  h. Claim made of better self-understanding
  i. Absence of desire for more psychotherapy
II. Interpersonal changes
  a. The patients' positive feelings for their therapists predominated and persisted
  b. An overall improvement in their relations, not only with some of the key people in their environment with whom they were involved in a major conflict but also with others
  c. Development of meaningful relationships with new people
III. Psychodynamic changes, from the observations of the evaluators
  a. Several patients had substituted various new and more adaptive defense mechanisms for those they had been utilizing
  b. The psychodynamic conflict underlying the patients' difficulties had been moderately or completely resolved in the majority of patients, and they were able to give examples that this had taken place. Thus, we suspected that psychodynamic changes had occurred.

Intrapsychic Changes

The question of symptomatic improvement requires discussion. It was clear that the patients had experienced only partial relief, but it was striking that their attitudes about their symptoms had changed. They did not seem to be overwhelmed by them any more. A patient said that his nervousness had "lost its kicks." A young man described it as follows: "I had a fear of lightning until I remembered that during thunderstorms my mother used to throw holy water around the house and talk about hell. I was so scared then, yet I had forgotten these episodes completely till I suddenly remembered them in one of my interviews. There it was. I was still a little nervous during last summer's hurricane, but it was nothing compared with my previous experiences." In general, then, there was a quantitative decrease in the intensity of the various symptoms which made them tolerable. They no longer seemed to interfere with the patient's overall functioning. One young woman put it this way: "My symptom has not been eliminated completely. I still get nervous at times. But now it is not crippling any more. I do not get paralyzed, as I used to, so I am able to do my housework." Another patient said that his depressive feelings were now "in bounds."

As mentioned before, the curious observation was made that the patients somehow did not want to abandon their symptoms completely because they were viewed as a solution. It was nice, so to speak, to keep them "in reserve." It may not have been the best alternative but it was, under the circumstances, the best the patient was able to come up with in handling his conflicts. This feeling of annoyance when someone appears to be in the position to offer a better solution has been repeatedly described already. The implication here is that the patient wants to keep things in his own hands, in his own house. He seems to say that deep inside he knows best. He wants his independence intact. The notion of "keeping the symptoms in reserve" serves the purpose to him of always having his old solution available in case some trouble arises in the future and the newly developed and somewhat shaky attitudes which have appeared as a result of the treatment might fail him.

It would be argued, as one may anticipate, that this observation might be used as documentation that short-term anxiety-provoking psychotherapy does not work. This is not the case. One should keep an open mind about newly acquired knowledge. Anxieties, depressions, obsessions, and so on, all are parts of our everyday lives, act as motivating factors and serve useful purposes as long as they are not too intense. Furthermore, there is an aspect of the repetition compulsion phenomenon or of conditioning in this unwillingness to part with symptoms completely. When a twenty-two-year-old college senior talked about it, he referred to his symptoms as "my familiar tricks." Familiarity is a way of avoiding anxiety. A thirty-eight-year-old woman, referring to her depression, put it as follows: "It was like an 'old shoe' to me. I had it for such a long time, so it is difficult to imagine life without it. It would be a pity to let it go completely; and, anyway, I don't think I can. But I am so glad that it is not so intense any more. This, for me, is a great relief." The symptom, then, seems to be an integral part of the patient's narcissism and is associated with the whole way he views himself. In this sense, it is also related to his self-esteem.

Self-esteem is greatly improved as a result of this kind of psychotherapy. The patient is less critical, less punitive, and less demanding. His attitude about himself has changed. However, if he needs to be critical or demanding of himself, he does it more appropriately, less indiscriminately. The improvement in self-esteem seems to be related to a decreased self-preoccupation and self-centeredness. Here is an example: "I used to blame myself whenever everything went wrong. It was all my fault. All my doing. Now I am not as self-critical. You know, I am not the center of the universe. I don't have that complex any more. When I make a mess of things now I say to myself, 'Okay, let's look at it and see.' I am capable of judging what is my own and what may be someone else's fault. I used to take the shuttle to New York. Every time the plane was late I blamed myself. I used to say, 'You should have taken an earlier plane, you should have woken up early,' followed by, 'It's my bad luck' and all that stuff. Now if the plane is late, it's late. It is due to the congestion at La Guardia, not my own fault."

A good way to assess improvement in self-esteem can be seen in changes in the patient's overall physical appearance, his degree of relaxation, his posture, and his facial expressions. All these can easily be observed during the interview and compared with the way he looked previously.

The change in the expectations, as a result of psychotherapy, is reflected in his more realistic appraisal of the disappointment in not obtaining "all that he expected from psychotherapy." Exaggerated expectations were viewed as poor motivating factors. In one way or another, however, most patients have expected to derive more from their psychotherapy than they actually admitted. Yet, in retrospect, I think they were better prepared to deal with whatever disappointments they felt. In general, they acted realistically. One patient admitted that in the back of his mind the thought had persisted that, as a result of psychotherapy, he should have learned to like engineering, the subject he was majoring in. "It was nonsense," he explained. "I know why I went into engineering and why I do not like it. I shouldn't have expected engineering to become as attractive as music has always been. I love music, but you can get more money out of engineering. Anyway you look at it — it boils down to that." The development of new attitudes has already been discussed briefly. This finding seemed to be predominant in the majority of the patients and it was related to another claim made by many: self-understanding. More about this later. As a result of being able to see his emotional problems in a different light, the patient was able to replace old attitudes, which he now was convinced did not serve their purpose, with new and more adaptive ones which seemed to provide him with tangible and immediate results.

There is another aspect of the patient's intrapsychic changes which has certain cognitive features. As already stated, we have been impressed by the patient's statements about "new learning" having taken place as a result of psychotherapy. This "new learning" did not seem to be so much an acquisition — such as a "new course," as one patient referred to it — of a new set of facts which the patient could utilize, but was a different kind of learning with an emotional dimension added to it which could be referred to as "emotional learning." If one were to introduce a new term into this jargon-ridden specialty of ours, the term "thymognosis" (Greek *thymos*, emotion or mood, plus *gnosis*, knowledge) may be appropriate, because it refers to both feeling and cognition. Whatever term one may use to describe it, however, new learning is what it is. In addition, it has another important aspect: problem-solving. This "new learning" also has novelty. Something unusual is experienced which the patient had not been aware of before — vast new possibilities appear on the horizon. Here again, self-understanding plays a dominant role. A technique of self-examination has been acquired which offers an unending potential for experimentation.

How much, then, is the patient's statement about new learning related to his wish to please the interviewer? Is he saying the things that his therapist would have wanted him to say?

TECHNICAL ASPECTS

The patients, in the follow-up interviews, were asked to give us concrete examples of new learning and problem-solving which occurred during therapy. More basically, considerable confidence was placed in the ability of the patient to use this "new learning" and "problem-solving" constructively in order to solve new problems or situations *after* therapy had been terminated. This, in our opinion, was the final and crucial test to prove that new learning had really taken place. Following is an example.

A twenty-five-year-old single woman, with impulsive sexual episodes which produced an illegitimate pregnancy followed by spontaneous abortion, had developed these difficulties during the time when she was nursing her dying mother and keeping house for her father. The therapy had centered on her relationship with her father. Her attachment to him, and her wish to be "his woman," was clearly understood. The sexual escapades were the results of thinly disguised incestuous wishes. After the therapy had ended she was seen in follow-up, during which she revealed that although she was now aware of her sexual impulsiveness and, therefore, had not been involved in any difficulties, she noticed that after her treatment had ended she had developed a tendency to overeat, which disturbed her because she had gained fifteen pounds in weight. She viewed this as a new problem. "So I tried to figure it out," she said; and then, becoming quite excited, she added, "It took some time, but I was determined I was going to get the answer. I questioned myself over and over about what made me go to the refrigerator and eat cookies between meals. It was when I kept on asking myself, 'Why do I eat cookies and why does nothing appeal to me?' that I finally decided to go to the refrigerator, very deliberately pick up a cookie, start to eat it, and let all thought that would occur to me at that time come streaming into my mind. And you know," she added triumphantly, "I got it! The first thing was not a thought, but the taste that the cookie produced. And then I suddenly remembered an episode when I was eight years old. My mother used to be a good cook and at Easter time she always baked some special Russian cake called 'paska.' I used to love it. That was the clue. I was just returning from school in the bus when I had a fight with my best friend, who made nasty remarks about my dress. It was a dress I loved, which my mother had made. We quarreled. She grabbed my arm, and she tore my sleeve. I was in tears. As I entered the kitchen I remember my mother sitting next to the stove. That wonderful smell of the freshly made 'paska' permeated throughout the room. I remembered that my mother put her arms around me. I cried and cried. Finally, to console me, she gave me a a piece of the cake, which was against the rules, because it had to be eaten on Easter Sunday only. Suddenly, the whole thing, the meaning of the cookies, became clear to me. I missed my mother so much. I burst into tears, and I cried for a long time. But I solved my own problem. I know now the meaning of the overeating." And, with tears in her eyes, she added, "This is why I am so grateful about my psychiatric treatment."

This kind of example shows clearly the ability of the patient to understand the void and depression which she felt about her mother's death, to utilize what she had learned in psychotherapy and put it into meaningful use, and to deal with her new problem — the overeating.

Technically, what the patient did is also of interest. The episode of the cookies, her letting her thoughts come in, paralleled the doctor's technique when he insisted upon getting all the details and associations available, to be used to explore and understand a specific behavior of the patient. Like putting all the pieces of the jigsaw puzzle together into a meaningful whole, which she had learned to do during her therapy, enabled this gifted young woman to solve her new puzzle.

Another patient talked about the problem-solving aspects of therapy in terms of discussing things with herself. This is how she described her therapy two years after its end. "I tried to remember what my doctor used to ask me. He had an accent and sometimes he would put things in a funny sort of way. It was kind of cute. Well, sometimes, I try to put the questions to myself exactly the way he used to ask them," and, imitating his accent, 'Come now, Mrs. B., are you definite that you are not exaggerating a tiny leetle beet?' I would say to myself. Well, that's what I do. It makes more sense, somehow, this way. I tried to answer him then in the same way I try to answer the questions I pose to myself now."

A critic may object. Isn't it possible that the patient is a mimic who imitates and parrots back the suggestions and statements made by his therapist? In my opinion this is not the case. The patient here does not repeat the words which he

has heard and does not understand, but on the contrary he
attempts to recreate the therapeutic atmosphere in order to
pose the questions needed for the solution of his problem.
The internalized dialogue which the patient utilizes reflects in
retrospect his relationship to the therapist, with whom he
identifies. This identification, in my opinion, is one of the
most essential first steps necessary for learning to take place.
It requires motivation, and it involves selectivity and
assimilation.

Experience with medical student teaching points to this
observation: unless they identify with their teacher of a
clinical subject, they have difficulty in learning. Anything
that interferes with this identification is actively avoided.[5]
For example, when we have had organized lectures and
seminars in psychiatry during the course of the students'
medical rotation, these exercises were boycotted by many of
the students, despite the fact that some of them were
interested in psychiatry. Those students who attended
admitted that they remembered very little from what transpired during these psychiatric sessions.

Interpersonal Changes

Since the therapist was considered partly responsible for all
these achievements, the patient's positive feelings for him
predominated throughout the course of psychotherapy,
persisted at its end, and continued long after. In another area
where we have observed changes, the development of new
attitudes on the part of the patient in his dealings with people,
as well as the attitudes of other people in reference to the
patient were significant. As has already been mentioned in the
discussion of the criteria for selection of patients, the ability
of the patient to have one meaningful relationship with
another person was emphasized and was considered important.
Because this relationship was scrutinized very carefully, it
provided us with a useful baseline to contrast with other
relations which were considered problematical for the patient.
It also offered us an opportunity to evaluate the changes in
the behavior of the patient which had taken place. Thus, the

documentation of change from the original attitudes and the replacement with new ones offers meaningful evidence that improvement in the interpersonal relations has taken place.

A thirty-year-old married man referred to a change in his relation to his father as a result of his treatment. He had always tried to please his father at the expense of his own wishes and constantly felt angry at his father for not demonstrating his love to him. This attitude had caused him a great deal of difficulty and was reflected in his poor performance at work. For example, although he would yield to his father, in whose business he worked, he was obsessed considerably by these emotions and, at times, procrastinated in his work so much he would sabotage the decisions reached between the two of them. After the end of psychotherapy he said he had learned that his problem was entirely his own responsibility rather than his father's, contrary to what he had originally thought. As a result of this, he now was able to discuss policy matters in the business quite openly and, on occasions, had disagreed with his father. He talked about a major expansion which had taken place as a result of his insistence, which turned out to be a successful venture from the business point of view. Although his father had originally objected to his suggestion, he had grudgingly given his consent and now was delighted by the turn of events. Thus, the improvement in his relationship with his father was reflected in his new attitude shown at work.

Tangible evidence of improvement in interpersonal relations has generally resulted in better work performance, academic achievement, or financial success.

Psychodynamic Changes

Usually the evaluators who saw the patients in follow-up interviews seemed to agree with them. There were certain areas, however, which the evaluators had to assess for themselves. The questions which were raised had to do with whether a dynamic change has taken place, whether a basic characterological improvement was accomplished, and whether the patient was parroting and imitating, or saying the things his therapist expected him to say. The answers to some of these questions are difficult. The evaluators must utilize a whole set of specific questions in an effort to test some of the answers the patients give them.

Malan has emphasized the importance of psychodynamic formulations for the assessment of the results of psychotherapy and has pointed to the difference between true psychodynamic improvements and improvements which he terms psychodynamically suspect.[6]

Psychodynamic change, in my opinion, involves a demonstration (as already mentioned) of substituting for various maladaptive defense mechanisms different ones which are more adaptive and are more useful to the patient in his dealings with others in his daily life. In addition, there must be a moderate or complete resolution of the psychodynamic conflicts. Resolution of a conflict does not always imply a clear understanding on the part of the patient of all the subtle ingredients involved in his original emotional conflict. At times, clear-cut indications on the basis of the patient's behavior outside the treatment hours, and the ability to deal with situations which previously were not manageable, point to clear-cut improvement and are a demonstration that psychodynamic change occurred quite consistently.

What was striking was the unusual number of patients who could verbalize quite clearly the various aspects of their emotional problem and talk about the resolution of this conflict in quite a sophisticated manner. There were some, however, who were not able to do so. An example of an unsophisticated response was found in a young man who had repeatedly used isolation and displacement of his anxieties when he was having emotional difficulties, had developed an incapacitating fear of animals in general and of cats in particular, and who was in constant quarrel with women. In follow-up he was only vaguely aware that this represented a displaced fear of his mother and sisters. He was, however, not only able to have a meaningful relationship with his girl friend but also enjoyed his new Jaguar sports car. Laughingly he said, "As you can see, Doctor, I love this big cat now." In sum, these changes occurred in our patients as a result of their psychotherapeutic work and not because of changes in their environment.

Long-Term Follow-up

In our controlled study it was of interest to note that by the end of the waiting period of the control patients who, of course, had not received psychotherapy, there was evidence of symptomatic improvement in somewhat less than half of these patients. This is a finding which other investigators have also observed and some have used as an argument that psychotherapy does not work. In a very few of the control patients there was also some change in self-esteem and in the expectations of the results of psychotherapy. A considerable number of these patients, while waiting, had taken various kinds of actions in an effort to solve their problems. In the majority they had not succeeded, however, and this had convinced them even more that they needed psychotherapy. A few patients thought that their actions did indeed help eliminate their anxiety and, although they realized the hit-or-miss aspect of their behavior, they were happy with the result and were not eager to pursue their plans for psychotherapy. Thus, out of the original thirty-six control patients, seven were lost at the end of the waiting period.

What was of interest, however, was that while, by the end of this waiting period, except for those mentioned above, no other changes had occurred in these control patients in comparison with the experimental ones, *after* these same patients received short-term anxiety-provoking psychotherapy *they compared favorably* with their experimental counterparts, and the intrapsychic, interpersonal, and psychodynamic changes already described occurred in the majority of both groups. In both groups the majority of the patients were utilizing what they had learned during psychotherapy to solve new emotional problems arising in their everyday lives. This was the most significant finding.

I am aware, of course, that only long-term follow-up will prove how durable these improvements may be, but, because of the mobility of the clinic population, many patients were lost because they moved away from the Boston area. For example, one-fourth of the experimental and control patients who had terminated their therapy were lost, and, despite our

Table 1. *Patients' Evaluation of Therapy*

Result	Controls (9)	Experimental (12)	Totals (21)	Approximate percentages
Moderate symptomatic relief	7	5	12	58
Improved self-esteem	8	9	17	82
New attitudes developed	8	10	18	86
New learning	7	9	16	77
Problem-solving	6	9	15	72
Use of problem-solving	5	8	13	62
Use of new learning	6	8	14	67
Self-understanding	9	10	19	91
Therapy successful	6	9	15	72
Overall change	8	10	18	86
Change in expectations	4	7	11	53
Improved interpersonal relations	9	7	16	77
Need of more therapy	1	5	6	28
Positive feelings for therapist	5	8	13	62

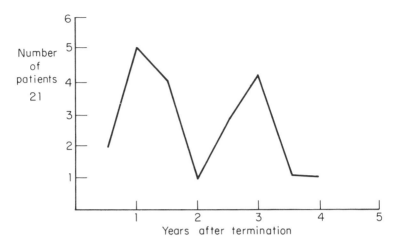

Time interval between therapy and follow-up questionnaire.

efforts, we could not track them down. In 1968 and 1969 we mailed questionnaires to thirty-four patients who participated in our controlled study and whose addresses were known. Twenty-one patients answered. Twelve were experimental, and nine were controls. They had terminated their treatment in anywhere from six months to four years previously. Table 1 gives their answers; Chart 1 shows the time interval between termination of therapy and follow-up questionnaire.

The numbers are small, but they reflect the overall trend of the follow-up findings already discussed. What seems to be significant is that although symptoms in one form or another persisted in nine out of the twenty-one patients (43 percent), at the same time five of these patients chose to rate their treatment as successful. Although six patients stated they wanted more therapy, four of these thought that the psycho-therapy was successful, and gave this as a reason for wanting to go on.

I wish again to draw attention to the continuous use of what was learned during psychotherapy in order to deal with and solve new problems after its termination. This occurred in 67 and 62 percent of the patients, respectively. Furthermore, the fact that eighteen patients (86 percent) thought that an overall change had taken place, and that sixteen (77 percent) had improved their interpersonal relations is also significant, because this points to the development of psychodynamic changes. Despite the fact that this follow-up study favors patients who were treated, as already mentioned, at the expense of those who were lost, nevertheless, in my opinion, these findings are encouraging.

At the present time, at the Beth Israel Hospital in Boston, we have set up a systematic study aimed toward evaluating the results of various kinds of psychodynamic psychotherapy, with every effort being made to specify criteria for effectiveness at the time of preevaluation interviews and to see the patients for as long as possible in follow-up interviews. We hope, then, to help demonstrate the usefulness of various kinds of short-term as well as other types of psychotherapy, to document the evidence adequately, and to contribute to the small but systematic efforts of those few investigators who think that for a great number of well-selected, but also quite incapacitated human beings, short-term psychotherapy is the treatment of choice.

We have also asked the patients to comment freely about their psychotherapeutic experience. Here is what a twenty-seven-year-old man, three years after the end of his treatment, had to say: "From time to time I can see a stressful situation coming on. I no longer avoid these circumstances, and to some degree I kind of look forward to them. Even though it may last for several days, I can look forward to greater self-understanding and to learning something new about life or myself almost every day."

A twenty-four-year-old single female patient, one year after her treatment ended, put it as follows: "My therapy helped me get through a very trying time and helped me understand what I was doing. Some specific behavior patterns changed. I don't sleep around any more, and I am able to make decisions based on my values rather than on my mother's," and then she goes on, "The attitudinal change, especially toward myself, was the greatest . . . I am much kinder to myself and hence to others. Dr. H. was great!''

All were not complimentary, however. Four years later, a twenty-five-year-old single woman wrote: ''Six months was too short a period for me. In addition, to be 'assigned' to a psychiatrist is ridiculous. Rapport with a therapist is very much based on compatibility of personalities. Please don't write me any more letters every year.'' Finally, two and a half years later, a twenty-one-year-old patient put it as follows in referring to his therapy: ''It made me understand the problems that had bound me up and made it difficult to make decisions. May I add that I am now in charge of a laboratory for one of the local chemical companies and I have gone back to college nights. Without treatment, I honestly feel that I would not have had the drive or self-confidence that is necessary to hold down a difficult job and go through college.''

These changes described by our patients speak for themselves. Although I cannot demonstrate convincingly nor offer a definite explanation about the therapeutic factors which may have contributed to the development of these changes and influenced the patients to make these statements, I suspect that the specific solution of the emotional problem, and the identification with the therapist, played a determining role. A critic may object, however. Is it possible that suggestion was more important? Is it possible also that the patient's willingness to play the therapist's ''game'' and his compliance to meet the therapist's expectations were just as crucial or even more important therapeutic parameters?

In my opinion the answer is no. It must be remembered that we do spend much time in evaluating and selecting our patients. We do not offer short-term anxiety-provoking psychotherapy to passive, compliant, and dependent individuals who sit back expecting that their therapist will do all the work and who accept readily what they are told. We do not view this kind of psychotherapy as a ''game'' that people play. On the contrary, we choose patients who are active, whose resistances are evidence of their character strengths and who despite their willingness to cooperate and participate in their treatment, nevertheless argue angrily at times, while on other occasions they get anxious after the confrontations of their therapists. If this anxiety is associated, as has been often suggested, with the fear of rejection by the therapist, or with the patient's inability to meet the expectations and goals of the therapist, why is it then that it appears only at times of clarification of the content of the emotional conflicts, or of the patterns of behavior which they have repeatedly tried to avoid? Why is it also possible that the patients dare to challenge their therapists when he introduces by mistake a subject or raises a question which appears irrelevant to them? I do hope, finally, that it will become apparent from reading the case material which follows that our patients are determined to understand themselves because they want to change.

PART III. CASE REPORTS

9

ANXIETY, FRIGIDITY, AND AGORAPHOBIA

Do Symptoms Protect Virtue?

A twenty-eight-year-old mother of an eight-year-old boy and part-time fashion model came to the psychiatry clinic because of anxiety, frigidity, and agoraphobia of three years' duration. During her evaluation she described her family atmosphere as happy while she was growing up. She was disciplined strictly by her mother, but she adored her father. She had an older brother and sister. Her mother was hospitalized when she was nine years old because of tuberculosis. During that time the girl was very close to her father, whom she described as an affectionate and loving man, and viewed herself as being "his pet." While her mother was away, her father spent most of his free time with the two girls. As she reminisced about her relation with her father she showed much feeling. She told about how he used to brush her hair and iron her dresses and exclaimed that he was both a father and a mother to her. She was jealous of her older sister and quarreled with her frequently. She described their encounters as "real female brawls."

Her mother returned from the hospital when the patient was fourteen years old. She claimed that she felt somewhat uneasy, but, for the sake of her father, she was happy to see her mother come back. She remembered that for the first time she took her sister's side in a family quarrel when her sister had a temper tantrum and struck her mother because she was so unhappy at the new family setup. The patient claimed to have been aware of this "uneasiness" because she had feared that her relation to her father was going to be interfered with from then on. It appears that she was also close to her older brother, but after he married and left she did not miss him very much. In high school she was an average student and enjoyed being very popular, in contrast with her sister, who hated school. She had many friends and dated a great deal. Her father was proud of her, but when she started to go out on "dates" he seemed to become unusually possessive and asked her questions about her various boy friends. He always tended to find fault with them.

She met her future husband while she was in high school. She soon fell in love with him and wanted to talk with her father about her plans to marry, but he became very angry, pounced upon the fact that he was a Catholic, and added, "No daughter of mine is going to get married outside our own church." She replied that the young man was willing to give up his church and be baptised as an Episcopalian, but her father was not appeased.

She married at the age of nineteen against the wishes of both of her parents. Her father refused to go to the wedding and did not even speak to her until after her son was born, one year later. Her mother was more sympathetic, although she also had disapproved because she felt that the girl was "too young" to be married.

Her symptoms of anxiety and frigidity appeared three years before she came to the clinic and had become progressively worse. Soon after the beginning of the frigidity she started to be afraid to go out alone and always wanted her husband to accompany her. This symptom, also, became progressively worse. Finally, she got tired of all this, wanted to do something about it, and consequently called to make an appointment at the clinic.

The patient was an attractive, intelligent woman who seemed eager to understand the causes of her symptoms. Although she claimed to be a part-time fashion model she was not as well dressed as one would have expected. During her evaluation interview she showed much affection for her father but also talked with warmth about her husband. She related well with the evaluating psychiatrist and expressed the conviction that she could get down to the bottom of all these problems which had turned her happy marriage into an unhappy one. The diagnosis was psychoneurosis with phobic features, and she was accepted for short-term anxiety-provoking psychotherapy.

It was thought that the emotional conflict underlying her anxiety and her frigidity was related to her early strong attachment for her father and subsequent guilt feelings at the time when her mother was away. The agoraphobia, however, loomed as more ominous. It was not clear whether this was associated to early dependent needs or whether it was related to her present difficulties with her husband as a result of her frigidity. It was thought, however, it was more likely that it was also related to this latter conflict.

In the first interview she came accompanied by her husband. She mentioned casually that she was afraid to leave the house without him; but, without waiting for the therapist to comment — which he was not prepared to do anyway — she started to talk about her quarrels with her sister when they were growing up and remembered angrily that when both her brother and her sister had announced their engagement her father gave his consent readily, while he was so inflexible concerning her own. She was obviously emotionally moved when she talked about her father's insistence that she give up her boy friend and of his not coming to her wedding. When she was asked why her father showed a different attitude in reference to their engagements, she blushed and answered, "Well, I was his pet, maybe?", and she continued, "And he always looked on me for help while my mother was away. When I told him about Bill and our future plans, he became so enraged that I thought he would hit me and said that we should wait for one year. I obeyed him, I waited all this time while I was working in his business. I tried to convince him to change his mind. Finally he agreed, but the day before the wedding he changed his mind. He could not accept the idea that I was going to be someone else's 'property.' He refused to come to the wedding, as you already know. I was very hurt. He did not speak to me from then on. It was at Christmas, one month after my son was born, when he called and said that he wanted us to go and visit him. He acted as if everything was all fine. Two months later he died of a heart attack. I felt crushed after his death. I could not believe that it was true."

The therapist asked her why she had not mentioned this fact during the evaluation interview. She answered that it had not crossed her mind at that time, and no one had asked her about it. She then added that at times she had a tendency to keep things to herself. The therapist insisted that she should be honest and straightforward during psychotherapy from this moment on. She wept as she continued to talk about her father's death, but she said she felt satisfied that they had made up with each other before he died. "It would have been terrible if he had died feeling angry at me, because he was a wonderful father and I loved him very much." The rest of the interview was spent in getting a detailed history, parts of which have already been described.

For the second interview she again came accompanied by her husband. This time the therapist decided to confront her with what she wanted to achieve during her therapy.

Doctor: Which one of your symptoms bothers you most — your fear of open spaces, your anxiety or your frigidity?

Patient: I hope all will go away.

Doctor: Not necessarily. Anyway, they won't go away. We must work to try to understand your problems.

Patient: It is hard to say. Somehow the fear of going out I can cope with, because my husband comes along with me.

Doctor: Just a minute. That is not coping with it. It is taking action without knowing what are the reasons for it. What about the frigidity?

Patient: This bothers me more. There is all this lying and pretending. You see, my husband does not know about it. I do a good acting job, but it bothers me. I think I would like to understand this problem even more. It makes me nervous.

Doctor: If so, what do you think it is associated with?

Patient: This is something which is hard to tell. (Then blushing:) It has to do with my parents. All this sexual education. My mother was very prudish.

Doctor: Are you, then, saying that it has something to do with your mother?

Patient: . . . Yes.

Doctor: So, if we tried to disentangle this aspect so that you could understand what it is all about, even if the fear of open spaces doesn't clear up, will you be satisfied?

Patient: Yes, Doctor.

At this point the patient changed the subject and mentioned that her husband wanted to know what she was talking about in her interview with me and added that since the previous interview she had been thinking a great deal about having been her father's favorite. She said, somewhat casually, that during the past week her sister had been admitted to a hospital for exploratory surgery and that she had to take care of her sister's five children. She then talked about her marriage. "I am happy up to a certain point. I make all the decisions on financial matters. I have learned to make decisions while living with my father at the time mother was in the hospital." She emphasized that there were many differences between her father and her husband and that she thought her father was really the better of the two men. She claimed to have learned to be independent while she lived with her father and again talked about having felt very disappointed in him when she found out that he disapproved of her husband. "I also decide about our having sexual relations," she said, "yet I don't want to give you the wrong impression." She paused for a while and then added that she had a sudden thought that maybe she married her husband just to spite her father. The therapist decided to pursue this issue out of the variety of topics the patient had brought up, because it seemed like a new realization, spontaneously arrived at on her part.

Doctor: Tell me more about that.

Patient: The thought just crossed my mind that maybe I was mad at him for something.

Doctor: What do you mean?

Patient: Maybe it was something that he had done to me way back.

Doctor: What do you have in mind?

Patient: Well, maybe it had something to do with the time I was growing up, and I was keeping house for him. After my mother came back from the hospital things went on exactly the same, but there was a difference in the air. Of course I was older then. I was fourteen.

Doctor: Are you saying that you were angry at your father, after your mother came back?

Patient: In a special sort of way. Yes. He wasn't the same with me as he had been before. He wasn't maybe as affectionate as I would have liked him to be.

She associated again to the conflict with her father and described at length the problems of her husband's religion and the anger that she felt toward her father during that time because she knew that he was not as religious a man as he pretended to be and was using his religion as a pretext. By the end of the hour the therapist was quite satisfied that the patient's relation to her father, at the time when her mother was away, had affected her relations with men in general and her husband in particular, especially in the area of sexuality, which seemed to be associated with the patient's frigidity. Because of this the therapist thought it was important to pursue this subject and try to keep the patient's interest confined to this area, either as it came up in the interviews in reference to past experiences or in terms of her transference feelings for him.

When the patient came for the next interview she was silent for a while, then she mumbled, "I haven't been honest with you, I gave you the wrong impression by telling you that I wanted to make all the decisions. I let you think the wrong thing and it bothered me that you got the wrong idea. I gave you the impression that I was an overbearing bitch with my husband."

Doctor: So you have some feelings about my impression of you?

The therapist here picks up the transference issue, since it was brought up also in the previous interview, and at that time he had not decided to pursue it.

Patient: Maybe, but I don't want you to have ideas that are not true about me.

Doctor: You don't want me to! You mean I do not have the choice of deciding for myself?

Patient (blushing): I suppose you have a point there. I never thought of it in this way.

Doctor: But isn't that what you do with your husband?

Patient: I thought of it more in terms of my father. You see, at the time when my mother was away at the hospital, I used to stay in the house a lot, particularly at night after my sister had gone to bed. We used to play card games with my father; we had much fun; but I always told him what to do, and he always did exactly what I wanted.

Doctor: So, as you were the boss with your father and with your husband, now you want to be the boss with me, here.

The therapist has a golden opportunity here in the early treatment to draw a parallel between the patient's feelings for two key men in her life and to the repetition of such feelings in the transference relation.

Patient: In a way, yes. I didn't realize this before. Throughout the week I have been thinking that I have given you the wrong impression and I felt compelled to change your mind about it.

Doctor: Compelled?

Patient (blushing again): Well, yes, but it isn't exactly true. For instance, I mentioned last week about sex. I take matters in my own hands, and one of the reasons is that my husband likes to do all the things that make me sick. I just couldn't stand it. When we have normal sexual relations, it's all right. This is very hard for me to talk about, it is very disagreeable.

Doctor: I understand. Go on.

Patient: I have never talked to anyone about this. I suspect that my husband likes other ways more than intercourse itself. I get so angry at him, I want to punch him. After we were married our sexual relations were pleasant and enjoyable. I used to have an orgasm quite often. But after two or three months my husband mentioned something about other ways, and I started immediately having a revulsion. Then I got pregnant and all this stopped for a while. I was so happy to have my little boy. From then on I have not enjoyed sexual relations. It leaves me cold. I don't want to show this to him because I'm afraid that it may lead into troubles between us — actually recently it has. It has caused a great deal of friction.

There was a long pause, and the patient's facial expression changed quite suddenly, her chin started to tremble and she turned pale. She mumbled, "My mother died that night! I felt so cold that night." There was a long pause.

Doctor: What do you have in mind?

Then suddenly she burst into tears and sobbed uncontrollably for quite a while. "I lied to you and to myself . . . " Finally, in a shaking voice, she revealed that just before her mother died she had telephoned the patient, asking her to drive over to pick her up and take her to work.

Patient: As I was getting ready to go, my husband asked me to have sexual intercourse with him. I felt guilty about having refused him so often before, so I hesitated, but I decided not to refuse him. I called my mother to tell her that I was too busy and that I couldn't drive her to work. She understood, because it had happened before. While we were still in bed, the chief of police, who was a friend of the family, called to say that my mother had been struck by a car as she crossed the street and had died instantly.

Doctor: You haven't mentioned all this before.

Patient: It just came to mind all of a sudden, and I couldn't lie any more.

Doctor: Do you think that this episode has anything to do with your frigidity?

Patient (bursting into tears again): I felt cold with my husband even before, as I told you. Not only did I feel cold, but I resented him and I thought about it before, but this time it was very different. It was as if his demands had something to do with my mother's death. I felt mad.

It is difficult to say at this point how much the patient had evaded. It was clear that this revelation was not unconscious, but in my opinion the spontaneity of the emotion associated with it was a new experience for her.

In the next interview she said that she had had a very busy week, with little or no time to do much thinking. She emphasized repeatedly that her husband wanted to know what was going on in her therapy. She said she did not want to tell him about it, however, for fear she might "spoil it or say the wrong thing."

Doctor: You mentioned this before. What do you think about talking to your husband about your psychotherapy?

Patient: It is not his business. I feel he is snooping.

Doctor: You want to keep it a secret?

Patient: In a way, yes. Particularly about what I talked about last week.

Doctor: What, specifically, do you mean?

Patient: You know . . . his being to blame, in a way, for my mother's death.

Doctor: He was not to blame. It was your choice.

Patient (in a tremulous voice): I don't like what you said.

Doctor: I know, but by your telling yourself that he was to blame, you pass onto him your own responsibility for your decision not to drive over for your mother. It makes it less painful for you that way, but it does not do any good, because you are not a little girl any more, and you are able to decide and to act. This is what you did. This was your choice.

The patient was silent for a while, and then she said that, although she had been quite upset when she learned of her mother's death, she had driven to the hospital alone. Her husband offered and insisted upon driving her, but she told him that she had to do it on her own. Then she went on to say, "I handle my son better now; I find it a lot easier to take care of him. You know, I still have my sister's children with me. She is back now and feels much better. I do get anxious, and it's a strain when I go outside. I have been feeling somewhat closer to my husband after our talks here." Soon after, however, her voice started to become tremulous again. Tears appeared in her eyes and she said, "The phone did ring actually while we were having intercourse, I confess this to you, I just couldn't say it the last time. I said it was afterwards, but actually it was during the time. I felt frozen. The chief of police told me that my mother was walking to the bus stop as the bus was ready to leave. She rushed across the street. Two young kids in a sports car were driving fast and failed to negotiate the turn. They hit my mother right at the bus stop. She died instantly. I felt so guilty.''

Doctor: I understand that this is very difficult for you, but confessing is not going to make things better. I am not your confessor. Now, there is another matter that I want to bring up. On the one hand you want to control me as you control your husband and father, and, at the same time, you view me as your confessor. I am here to help you unravel your own emotional problems. Now tell me, is there anything more in all this?

Patient: This is hard. Why do you make me do this?

Doctor: I don't make you do anything. I just think there is something else that bothers you. Why were you feeling guilty?

Patient: Because I chose my husband over my mother.

Doctor: This was a matter of choice. Maybe it was the wrong choice. But why guilty? Guilty implies a crime — one pleads guilty or not guilty to a crime. What was the crime, Mrs. R.?

Patient (long pause and looking very tired): I told you last time that I have not enjoyed sexual relations. It is not true. I did enjoy intercourse very much. I was angry at my husband only when he wanted me to do these other things. That day when we had sexual intercourse the normal way I remember that I was enjoying it just before the telephone rang, but I did not have an orgasm, Doctor. That's the honest truth. Telling you these things makes me feel very queer.

Doctor: Queer?

Patient: It means it is a kind of worrying feeling — the same things that brought me here to the clinic. It is the same feeling that comes over me when I go outside. I have never enjoyed sexual intercourse since that time. You were right, Doctor.

Doctor: But what was queer about it?

Patient: Well, that is not the exact word. Maybe it's anxiety.

Doctor: You said "queer."

Patient: It's so sad, yet I feel giggly inside when I'm telling you all this.

Doctor: So it has something to do with me?

Patient: Hmm . . . yes. I mean, no.

Doctor: You mean yes.

Patient: Like seeing you as my father or my husband. We already talked about this.

Then she turned pale and was quiet for some time.

This acknowledgment of the transference seemed to open the doors for more significant recollections from the past which continued also in the following interview.

Doctor: What are you thinking about?

Patient: . . . I don't know how to say this! . . . It just came to my mind just now, out of the blue. I had forgotten about it, yet I knew it all along. I lied to you. (Then sobbing:) There was my poor mother lying dead on the cold pavement while I was having an orgasm. I shall never forgive myself.

Realizing that the time was approaching for the end of the interview, she was able to pull herself together and say, "I wasn't able to cry that time. I felt frozen. I knew what was happening and I understood immediately what the chief of police was trying to tell me. At my mother's funeral I cried a bit, but it was somewhat forced. I felt that I was really putting on some kind of a show. This made me feel even worse, because I was quite close to my mother. She and I had some good times together, particularly before she got sick. I used to play with my dolls while she was knitting. She also used to tell me nice stories. She was strict, but she was also a good mother."

At the following interview she said that her husband had accompanied her. She talked at length about various episodes of her childhood and about the closeness between herself and her mother. She then again started to cry.

Patient: Why is it I could not cry then?

Doctor: I wonder what was in your mind at that time?

Patient: I kept on thinking, if I cry, if I am weak, what would people think?

Doctor: People?

Patient: Yes.

Doctor: Whom do you have in mind?

Patient: Oh, my sister, my aunts, all those people at the funeral.

Doctor: Whom do you have in mind in particular?

Patient: . . . You mean?

Doctor: I mean nothing. I am asking you. I don't know.

Patient: It's my father . . . I don't know why I did not want to admit it. It was there in my mind and I knew it, but I just couldn't tell you when you asked.

Doctor: You know, Mrs. R., you lie just to cover up looking at yourself and at your feelings. Then you confess and think that all is forgiven. Is this what you did with your father?

Patient: In a way, yes. I had to cover up my feelings to show my father that I had a special feeling only for him. How could I admit that I loved my mother when I took her place? How could I admit this to him? Do you understand? I had to lie?

Doctor: Even after she died?

Patient (sobbing): Oh, no!

Doctor: I know that you loved your mother, but it was difficult for you to accept these feelings when you had special feelings for your father at the same time. Then, of course, there was also this episode on the day when your mother died.

Patient: Yes, I know.

She continued to talk, showing much emotion about her mother. Often she was in tears. It appeared that she seemed to be grieving for the first time about her mother's death. No attempt was made, therefore, to interfere with his spontaneous and therapeutic catharsis.

With the grieving out of the way, as expected, the transference reappeared as the major issue.

The next time there was a striking change in her appearance. She was dressed in a beautiful dark suit and was wearing high heels. She smiled broadly but announced that she had felt unusually apprehensive about coming to the clinic. It developed that when her girl friend, who was supposed to drive her over, changed her mind at the last minute, she insisted that her husband change his plans and accompany her. He agreed reluctantly. She smiled and added that although she thought she was getting better, she found herself getting sick all over again. Then, continuing to smile, she said, "I saw you walking down the corridor talking to that pretty girl. Is she a doctor? or a student? or something like that?"

Doctor: Why do you ask?

Patient: I know there are a lot of people who get their training here. I'm sorry. I didn't mean to be nosey.

Doctor: Tell me more about your feelings of being nosey.

Patient: You see I was walking behind you. You didn't see me. You seemed to be enjoying talking to her. Both you and she were laughing. I couldn't hear what you were saying, and I felt a little embarrassed because I was walking close by. I turned to my husband and said, "See, there is my doctor." He said, "Why don't you introduce me to him?" I got angry and told him, "Can't you see that he is busy?" He said he did not think that you were that busy if you were talking to a pretty blonde. I was mad at him. This is the kind of thing about him which always annoys me. He has no understanding of things. He's so uncouth.

Doctor: You seem to be unusually annoyed at your husband.

Patient: Yes. (Emphatically:) He had no business talking to you.

Doctor: You also, somehow, wanted to protect me from him? Why should that be?

Patient: Oh, no. I didn't want to protect you. If anything, I was a little — well, I don't know how to put it — (blushing) kind of annoyed at you. It was the same feeling I had on Sunday. You see, Bill and his wife came over to visit us, and we had a good time, but I felt for the first time somewhat uneasy with Bill. I don't know how to describe it, but it was somewhat the same feeling seeing you in the corridor. I was feeling queer all over.

Doctor: There we go with that "queer feeling" again.

Patient: You know, I thought Bill looked very attractive, and — come to think of it — I had sex on my mind; but, you see, after they left, my husband went to sleep. I watched television all night. I saw the late late show, and I remember seeing a very good movie. It was all about love.

Doctor: So, love seemed to be very much on your mind.

Patient: The thought occurred to me, maybe it was a mistake to marry my husband.

She continued to talk at length about her husband's faults, and then she added, "Maybe my father was right. My father was so good to me and I took such good care of him when my mother was in the hospital, but I'm not a good wife to fath . . .

Doctor: To your *father?*

Patient (blushing): Oh, My God, I meant to say my husband.

Doctor: Yes, I know, but you said father.

Patient: I guess so if that's what I said —

Doctor: You mean you have forgotten?

Patient: Well, no.

Doctor: That is exactly what you said, even if you did not exactly finish the word, so what about it?

Patient: You know what I mean.

Doctor: No. As a matter of fact, let us try to see what you've been telling me today. You talked about the same queer feeling that you had when you saw me in the corridor talking with a blonde as you had for Bill. You talked about sexual thoughts and about your doubts in reference to your husband. Finally, you talked — by mistake, of course! — about being a good wife to your *father.* Now let us look at what all this means.

The therapist by recapitulating focuses the patient's attention in the underlying sexual wishes for her father.

Patient (still blushing): I guess I must have had some feelings of that kind, way back then. I remember now. When my mother was in the hospital I used to cook for my father and he used to say, "You cook so well, you cook better than your mother." And I would get that warm feeling inside like being a wife to him.

Doctor: So you see that some of the feelings that you have for other men are the same that you had for your father at that time; but, for one reason or another, you seem to exclude your husband. Why is that?

Patient: Only since the time my mother died. Up to that time, as I told you, everything was all right between us.

Doctor: I know, but do you think that maybe your

mother's death had something to do with your wanting to be a wife to your father?

Patient (pauses for a long time and then says): God forbid, not in *that* way, I never thought of it. (Seeming to be very upset, finally:) I don't want to think about it.

Doctor: It's time you thought about it, if you want to understand yourself.

Despite the expectation an angry response, the therapist continues to focus in the area of the main conflict.

The patient glared back, but it was the end of the hour.

As a reaction to this difficult interview one may expect some sort of an attempt on the part of the patient to avoid the issues which had been discussed.

She came ten minutes late next time, and as soon as she sat down she started to cry. She said that she had felt very discouraged during the week. She was sure she was sliding backward. She had felt restless and upset and could not keep her eyes open. Then she said, "I felt guilty about having thoughts about enjoying sex. This is something I discovered here with you when I remembered having an orgasm that day when my mother died. But then you brought up the idea that I wanted to be a wife to my father."

Doctor: You did. It was *you* who brought it up. I put it more succinctly.

Patient: I know. I thought about it. It doesn't do any good to blame others. It was because I remembered all these feelings during the week that I was feeling so restless; but, deep inside, I know you're right. (Seeming to relax, and then with a smile:) My husband hasn't touched me, he hasn't come close to me for weeks. I have an awful feeling when I go outside. I'm frightened. Monday, when I had to go to the supermarket I was terrified I would do something foolish.

Doctor: Foolish?

Patient: Faint or something, like dropping something or receiving . . .

Doctor: What do you mean?

Patient: Maybe people would look at me. Whatever I try to do isn't right. My husband isn't happy, and I feel tense. I feel like running away from things. I feel frustrated, and it takes me five minutes to quiet down.

Doctor: "Guilty," "enjoyed sex," "your husband hasn't touched you," "you want to do something foolish." You discovered all these things here? What are you trying to tell me?

Patient: My husband is not coming close to me. Maybe this has upset me more than I thought. He leaves me alone. The thought occurred to me, "Maybe with someone else . . . (blushing) I have been thinking about it all week. That's why I have been so upset.

Doctor: Here is finally the real reason!

Patient: I feel so faint, maybe I'll pass out right here. If I faint, I'm helpless.

Doctor: Tell me about it.

Instead of supporting the passive helpless position the therapist continues his anxiety-provoking probing.

Patient: The two feelings are very different. The first one is the one I already mentioned to you — the queer feeling that has to do with being frustrated, but then it is this other feeling which makes me feel scared. It is a scary feeling that makes me weak and dizzy, and then I am afraid I may faint.

Doctor: What will happen if you faint?

Patient: . . . I collapse. I fall down, you know . . .

Doctor: Yes, I know, go on.

Patient: Nothing else, I faint . . .

Doctor: What happens when you faint?

Patient: I lie down on the cold ground.

Doctor: Yes —

Patient: Hmm . . . (looking very pale).

Doctor: Come on, what do you have in mind?

Patient: It is what will happen to me when I am lying down that worries me.

Doctor: On the cold pavement . . . ?

Patient: Oh, no, you know . . . it is that . . . I can't resist!

Doctor: Resist?

Patient: Yes, maybe somebody will take advantage of me.

Doctor: Whom do you have in mind?

Patient: I'm noticing this queer feeling right now. (Then, adding quickly:) No, not you! The same thing happened to me when I was buying meat at the counter the other day. There is a butcher whom I have known for a long time. He's a nice guy, but he is of a different religion.

Doctor: Hmm!

Patient: Well, he's Catholic, see?

Doctor: Hmm.

Patient: This religious issue seems to be very important.

Doctor: You seem to be telling me something.

Patient: You see, my father *is* Protestant.

Doctor: Yes, I know; but what does your father have to do with it?

Patient: Doctor, are you teasing me?

Doctor: No, I am not. I want to know what you have in your mind.

Patient (long pause): He is short and my father *is* tall. They don't look at all alike.

Doctor: Do you have to choose someone who is so different just to avoid thinking of your father in this way?

Patient: It's so horrible.

Doctor: There is nothing horrible about it if it's the truth. Anyway, your father is dead. He is alive only in your own mind.

Patient: Deep inside I know that this is the way it is, but it is so — so queer.

Doctor: It is this "queer feeling" that we know so well by now. There is something also, however, that maybe you thought of. Do you realize that this fear of open space and of going out actually protects your virtue and keeps you faithful to your husband?

Patient: Is that what it is? I never thought of it in that way!

During the next interview the patient announced that she had discussed at length her psychotherapy with her husband. "You know what he said? He said I was crazy. He was also hurt when I told him I hadn't been satisfied. He was surprised, because he thought that I was not interested in sex, which was true, and that he was abstaining just for my sake. Later on that night we had relations. It was not too good. It's hard to accept a notion of enjoyment of sex, but I know it will take some time to work all these things out.''

Doctor: Yes, I agree.

Patient: Anyway, the other fellow is married.

It seemed to be time to pull things together and make connections between the patient's symptoms and her sexual desires.

Doctor: Let us recapitulate what we know. There were your feelings for your father while your mother was sick in the hospital, which we know so well by now. Then, when your mother returned, you felt disappointed in him and things were not going to be the same any more. You challenged your father by marrying a man whom he did not like. You enjoyed sexual relations at first, but because of your guilt at the time of your mother's death you started feeling frigid and you eliminated your husband as a sexual partner from then on. Soon you became frustrated, and you developed symptoms of fearing to go out and of wanting your husband to go out with you; yet, at the same time, you had the wish to go out to faint and for someone to take advantage of you. Your phobia was a way to protect your virtue from your sexual desires for these other men. Who is this other man? Someone who is as different from your father as he could be, someone like your husband. Now, all this time you have your husband at home, the man whom you chose and with whom you had satisfaction in sexual relations; but, instead, you are looking at other men.

She was quiet for a long time, and then she said, ''I have been thinking this past week of going back to work. You know, I used to be a singer and a pretty good one. I used to do some part-time fashion modeling up to two years ago. I enjoyed it very much, but I gave it up when I had to sing in front of ladies' groups because I was self-conscious. Women are more critical than men. They expect a great deal from you. I remember I overheard one woman say once, 'She's not so hot.' She thought she was better than I. Women are always very critical and jealous.''

Doctor: Whom do you have in mind particularly?

Patient: Well, my husband, I suppose.

Doctor: Is it possible at times that you view your husband as a woman when you want to control him and when you are an "overbearing bitch" with him, as you have told me? But let us not forget that he is very much of a man and not a woman. Who comes to your mind?

Patient (hesitating): Women over forty, you know . . . settled women.

Doctor: Like whom, for example?

Patient: I have been trying to avoid it — but I know — I know it is my mother.

Doctor: I understand.

Patient: I should not avoid these feelings. After all the work I have done here I must learn to live with them, but it isn't easy.

Doctor: Yes, we have looked into the guilt feelings for your mother. We also know that you felt competitive with your mother in the past. Now we know that these feelings exist at present. I know it is difficult because you loved your mother. But I do think that you are ready and able to stand on your own two feet. Of course, you must prepare yourself for future difficulties of this kind. Furthermore, you are going to be anxious when you sing before all those "settled" ladies.

Patient: I know that I don't have to worry so much about criticism from women. As a result of my work here I can stand on my own two feet now, but I know I'll be anxious.

Doctor: It seems to me that we have worked on what we agreed upon quite well. Do you think that we should think about finishing treatment?

Patient: I have been thinking about it, also. If I go back to part-time work it would be difficult to come over here. Maybe it wouldn't be such a bad idea, although I know I shall miss these sessions.

Doctor: I understand. I'll see you in two weeks, then.

The patient returned in two weeks, to say that all was going well. She described how she had sung in front of a group.

Patient: I felt a little anxious when I appeared in front of a group. There must have been two hundred women. I kept

165

thinking of all I had discovered here. It was like rehearsing, preparing myself. This way helped a great deal. It was one of the local club meetings. I told myself at the time I was anxious, "Think of what you talked about with the doctor. Look what you have learned." And it all seemed to help a great deal. I calmed down, and from then on I was able to sing very well. The worst part of this was the day before; but, after all, you must feel kind of anxious in order to perform well. After it was all over I felt fine. I'm planning to go to work tomorrow.

Doctor: What about your husband?

Patient: He thinks I'm much better. I'm less tense, we talk a great deal, and we have had intercourse seven times in the last two weeks. I told him I wanted him to take the initiative, and he did. It has been much better. I don't want to be the boss any more. I am tired of being an "overbearing bitch." The first two times it was much more enjoyable, but I did not have an orgasm. Afterwards I felt much better about all this. Two days ago I had an orgasm for the first time in three years. I didn't like the idea of being frustrated. I kept on thinking of all we talked about, and it makes sense. I think it finally sank in, and now I feel better . . . My boy is doing well in school.

Doctor: What do you think about stopping the treatment, then?

Patient: I have been thinking about it, Doctor. I'm ready for it. I think I can try to figure out my future problems. I feel quite confident; but I'll miss you, Doctor.

Doctor: I also think that you can figure out things in the future if you continue to do the hard work you have demonstrated you are able to do here so well.

Patient: Thank you very much.

A year later the patient was seen in a follow-up interview. She said that she had felt somewhat anxious at times, but in general her relationship with her husband had been good and her agoraphobia had disappeared. She felt that she was using what she had learned in psychotherapy, particularly at a time when a man had fallen in love with her. She admitted that she was interested in him, but she was able to handle the

CASE REPORTS

situation fairly well because she was happy with her husband. "I felt anxious for a while and thought of talking to my husband about it. But then I decided that it was up to me and that I could solve my problem alone. From then on, it was not too hard any more."

Seven years later the patient called to say that she was fine, except that her husband had some difficulties with his boss. She asked for the name of a private psychiatrist for him.

Doctor: So you are still the boss?

Patient: Oh, no, no . . . well, maybe just a little.

All was well. She had another child — a boy, aged four.

Discussion

The psychodynamics of this case may be obvious, but let us briefly recapitulate. The patient's anxiety was associated both with her frigidity and with the agoraphobia. Partial repression and conversion gave rise to the frigidity, and isolation, displacement, and projection produced her phobia. It was this latter symptom which brought her to the clinic, but she chose to resolve the former in the beginning of her treatment because, in my opinion, it was easier for her to deal with it. She knew, of course, that it was partially related to the sudden and traumatic death of her mother about which she sooner or later had to talk. She was unaware, on the other hand, of the implications of her agoraphobia.

After she was able to grieve and acknowledge to herself her love and competition for her mother, she felt better, but neither the frigidity nor the agoraphobia disappeared. She was now ready, however, to make an effort to resolve the emotional conflicts underlying these two symptoms, and it was of interest that she used her transference feelings for the therapist to make the transition.

Her frigidity served a double purpose. It was a way to ward off her husband and, at the same time, to keep her unresolved incestuous wishes for her father alive. The agoraphobia, of course, protected her virtue whenever her strong heterosexual desires pressed for expression as they did, for example, in the episode with the Catholic butcher.

It may appear that everything went a little bit too smoothly in this case. Yet in retrospect, it is hard to portray the internal struggle this woman was experiencing in bringing her feelings into the open, despite the fact that she was most of the time aware of some of them. The therapist encouraged her to bring her positive feelings for her father and her mother into the therapeutic situation. The transference feeling for him predominated and helped her to see for herself how her old conflicts were repeated in her daily life and, at the same time, to recognize the methods she used to handle them.

Technically speaking, the role of the doctor was to raise anxiety-provoking questions and try to tie things together for her. It was the patient who was able to work hard, both inside and outside psychotherapy, and as a result of this, she was ready to terminate her treatment early. The success of her psychotherapy depended entirely upon her own efforts.

10

ANXIETY AND HOMOSEXUALITY

A Cover Up?

A twenty-one-year-old male college student decided to seek psychiatric help because of his feelings of nervousness associated with his homosexual tendencies of several years' duration. What precipitated his visit to the clinic was a recent episode involving his reluctantly agreeing to go out on a double date at the insistence of a friend. After the dance, while his friend was "making out" with his own girl friend, the patient had a sudden urge to run away; but he sat, frozen, in the back of the car while his date made some derogatory remarks about his masculinity. After this episode, he felt both angry and nervous and he could not sleep. The next day, when his friend criticized him for being cold with his date and for embarrassing him by not being "a man," he felt most uncomfortable and started to blame himself for being a coward. This anxiety increased. During the next few weeks he was unable to concentrate, and his grades started to suffer. When one of his tutors warned him about his poor academic performance and implied that if this continued he might fail in his major courses, he became alarmed. In this state of emotional crisis he decided to seek psychiatric help.

He traced his difficulties back to the time of his puberty, when he noticed for the first time that women did not arouse him. On the contrary, he had felt a certain "vague interest" and "general fondness" for boys. He said that he had been afraid of, and had stood in awe of older men; but he admitted that, on some occasions, he had engaged in mutual masturbation with two younger boys when he was twelve and fourteen years old. He denied having overt homosexual relations and mentioned that, on occasion, he had dated girls. Actually, when he was sixteen he did associate with a girl who was two years his senior, but she soon became seriously ill and died a few months later. He was very upset after this event, and when another girl in high school showed an interest in him, he avoided her because he was frightened that she also might die.

There were five members in his family. He had an older brother and a younger sister, and he described the family relations as close, but strained. His father, a lawyer, was in his early fifties. "He irritates me because he is so intolerant of other people's mistakes, including his sons'! He sits there and judges you instead of giving you a chance to defend yourself." Slowly he became unable to communicate with his father; but he did not show his feelings because he was conscious of a vague need to be protected by his father, although he could not understand why this should be. He experienced the same reactions in his relations with his older brother, whom he considered an unimaginative and rigid individual, but whose protection he also sought. He said that they quarreled on occasion.

He was very close to both his mother and his sister. His sister, who was four years younger than he, had married when she was fifteen years old and lived in California. He said he missed her very much. He described his mother as young, demonstrative, understanding, and very beautiful. He repeated that he loved his mother very much. As soon as he mentioned this, a smile appeared on his face, and when the interviewer commented on it, he said that he was amused by the thought that his mother was always in his room complaining of the mess in there and straightening out his bed. He added, however, that he felt rejected by his mother because she would always praise his brother for keeping his room clean and, on occasions, she would take his brother's side when the two of them had an argument.

During the ages of five and twelve he was quite obese, which the other children teased him about. When he was eight years old he injured his left leg in a fall from his sled. He said that he did a great deal of crying and was taken care of by his father, who was solicitous toward him. "He sat next to my bed and stroked my leg, saying that it would make the pain go away. I stayed in bed for a whole week and my dad used to tell me stories," he said. At that time he felt that his father loved him and wanted to protect him for the rest of his life. He contrasted this attitude with that of his mother, who said that if he were a man he shouldn't have cried so much. This had made him very angry.

During puberty he changed, and from then on he was more attached to his mother and more antagonistic toward as well as afraid of his father. He had many friends of both sexes, and his academic performance in high school was superior. Although not athletically inclined, he was president of the school debating club. After he graduated with honors he went to college, where he described himself as being very popular. He had several male friends, but he considered himself as being shy with girls. He repeated that his "homosexual tendencies" began during puberty. It was then that he started to masturbate, always having a fantasy of performing "frontal intercourse with a boy who turned out to be built like a girl and who wore a beautiful dress." He was vague about this when asked to give more details.

During the interview he spoke freely and had easy access to his feelings about all the members of his family. He interacted well with the interviewer and showed a considerable degree of flexibility and inquisitiveness.

He was a good-looking, friendly, bright, and curious young man, well motivated to overcome his anxiety and understand his "homosexual problem" which interfered with his wish to be married eventually and raise a family. He said that he had taken a part-time job to pay for his psychotherapy, if he was found to be acceptable by the clinic, because he did not want to borrow the money from his mother.

After the end of the evaluation it was thought that he fulfilled our criteria for selection. The psychodymanic hypothesis of his difficulties suggested that his homosexual tendencies were defensive in nature and served the purpose of keeping him close to his mother, and that his feelings of antagonism for his father and brother resulted from competition with them for his mother's affection. At the same time, he felt rejected by his mother, and this gave rise to the need to be protected by his father. The solution of this dilemma which he had devised was to stay away from women and be interested in men. In general, his life appeared to be essentially an asexual one. The prediction was made that, if he was helped to become aware of this emotional conflict in relation to his transference feelings for the therapist he would be able to solve his problem, with the result that his sexual interest in men would decrease and at the same time he would be able to have dates and relate to women, which, it was thought, he was fully capable of achieving.

During a goal-setting interview he was told that he was accepted for psychotherapy, which was going to be of short duration, and an effort would be made to help him understand the basic problems that brought him to the clinic. He agreed readily.

He started his treatment by talking critically about his mother because of her not being sympathetic with some of his views. He remembered, for example, that when his mother was pregnant with his sister, when he was four years old, he used to run around the chair in which his mother was sitting, asking her a lot of questions and occasionally tapping her on the abdomen and asking why it was so big. He remembered her smiling and telling him not to be silly. At times, she said, "Don't do this, it might hurt the baby inside." He could not understand what she meant because he could not see any baby. On one occasion, he jumped suddenly on his mother's lap. She screamed and pushed him off, saying that he had hurt her. He fell on the floor, cut his arm, and cried for a long time, but got no sympathy from his mother. When she came back from the hospital he was angry with her and hid under the bed. "She had a rough time trying to find me."

His temper tantrums increased from then on. He remembered

his mother mentioning that he had changed after the birth of his sister and, on one occasion, threatening to send him away. He switched the subject abruptly and talked about being terrified at the thought of being a homosexual. "It would be a terrible thing." He again spoke about his fantasy of his having "frontal intercourse with a boy who had the appearance of a girl".

Doctor: Could you give me some details?

Patient: There is something peculiar about the boy's clothes. The boy is never naked. I don't see his face. There is something about a woman's dress which he wears. Women's clothes offend me and make me feel cold all over. When I see a girl I feel as if I'm hurt.

Doctor: Hurt?

Patient: Yes; it is as if someone grabbed me by the arm and threw me in the trash.

Doctor: You mean, as when your mother threatened to send you away?

Patient: Yes, exactly. I told you that I love my mother, but I am also afraid of being hurt by her. I used to have tantrums, but I also enjoyed being forgiven by my mother. In the beginning I felt that both my parents loved me, but after my sister's birth I had the feeling that nobody cared for me. I had many temper tantrums then in order to draw attention. My mother used to get so angry! She used to say, "What is going to become of you"? After that I would go and ask her to forgive me and I would try to please her, but I felt always irritated inside.

Doctor: You said the same thing about your father.

Patient: I always try to be nice nowadays, and I can't bear arguments any more. I used to be different, however. I was jealous of both my brother and my father. I tried to get my mother's affection and draw her away from them. It was always this way after I was twelve years old.

Doctor: I am confused. When were you close to your father and when did it change?

Patient: Well, it is like this. I was close to my mother, but after my sister was born I was mad. Then I wanted my father's protection when I was twelve, and had all these homosexual wishes. After that I became angry at my father and my brother, and again I was close to my mother, but I still feel that she may reject me.

At this point the therapist thought it was time to clarify the issues to be dealt with in psychotherapy.

Doctor: Now, it seems, we have to decide at this point what you want to achieve in psychotherapy. As I understand it, it is your so-called homosexual desires you want to get rid of. We must, therefore, try to see how they have developed, what they really do signify, and what they are related to.

Patient: So-called homosexual?

Doctor: Yes. After all, homosexual is a word which means "of the same sex." What is of importance is to see in what way your relations with men and women have developed as you were growing up, in what way they have interfered with your present life. Words or labels are just descriptive and do not serve the purpose of understanding your feelings.

Patient: I see. You mean I may not be a homosexual?

Doctor: No. It means that I do not know. Now are these anxious feelings of yours particularly associated with your father and brother or with your mother?

The therapist here is unwilling to reassure the patient and relieve his anxiety.

Patient: The cold feeling has to do with my mother. It is this hurt feeling that I have when I go out with girls. This feeling is the same when I think I am a homosexual, and it is this which makes me anxious. My feelings for my brother and my father are different.

Doctor: In what way?

Patient: I am angry with them but I don't show it.

Doctor: What feelings do you want to get rid of?

Patient: The anxious feelings about being a homosexual which are vaguely connected with my mother.

Doctor: Okay. Let us concentrate in this area, and try to understand where these anxious feelings come from.

In the next interview he started to talk about work. He had a part-time job at an insurance company where there were many girls, and he said that sometimes he was interested in them, but always several at a time; and he continued, "But every time I think of a girl in particular I start feeling frightened. It is that same feeling of being hurt inside. And to get away from it I start thinking about guys and I feel better."

Doctor: Can you describe these feelings that you have for the girls and for your mother?

Patient (looking puzzled): I don't know how to put it.

Doctor: In what way, do you think, are these feelings of yours about women associated with your homosexual tendencies?

Patient: I don't know; but I want to do everything I can to get rid of these feelings.

Doctor: Don't forget that the answer must come from you. Now tell me more about your mother.

Although earlier a tentative agreement had been reached between the patient and his therapist on the emotional problem to be solved during the treatment, on the basis of the information available, it now appeared that the focus should be more on the understanding of his feelings about women and the ensuing conflicts rather than on the homosexuality which was the patient's original complaint.

Patient: My mother is a stunning redhead. I always had an admiration for older women! I remember when I was young I was quite interested in how women are built and I read a lot of books about art and some about sex. But after a while my parents discovered them and took them away from me.

Doctor: Your parents?

Patient: Yes.

Doctor: Who in particular?

Patient: Both of them.

Doctor: Come now, who in particular?

Patient: You know, uh — (hesitatingly) . . . my mother.

He was silent for a while, but then he continued to describe his fondness for his mother. He said that when his father and his brother were not at home, he enjoyed being alone in the house with his mother. "She is usually in the kitchen, and we talk about one thing or another and the time flies. After a while, usually, I start feeling guilty and I have to leave and go up in my room and read."

Doctor: What are you guilty about?

Patient (blushing and ignoring the question): I read either an anatomy book or those magazines about sex — *Playboy*, stuff like that.

Doctor: I thought your mother took them away.

Patient: Oh, that was when I was young.

Doctor: And now?

Patient: Oh, my mother knows about them. The other day she told me that she did not like very much the girl on the October issue of *Playboy*. When I asked her why, she was embarrassed and said that she thought the girl was too well developed on top.

Doctor: On top?

Patient: That's what she said initially. (Irritably:) You know she meant her breasts.

Doctor: You seem to be annoyed by my questions.

Patient: Well, you go into all these details.

Doctor: Can you tell me how you feel right now at my questions?

Patient: Damned mad.

Doctor: Because I inquire into what you and your mother talk about?

Patient: In a way, yes. It is the same feeling that I have when my brother or my father comes in when I am with my mother. They interfere.

Doctor: So, I interfere, too!

Patient: I know that you have to ask questions, but that's how I feel. It's like being punished.

Doctor: Okay. No one is punishing you. But you say you feel guilty when you spend too much time in the kitchen with your mother. Then you feel as if I am punishing you. Now what about all this?

Patient: I don't know. There isn't really much to say.

Doctor: The time is late, but you must think about all this. We must stop now.

The transference issue is picked up, even if the feelings for the therapist are negative. The patient seemed relieved as the hour ended.

The next time he announced that there had been some trouble at home over the weekend. He had a quarrel with his brother because he had trampled on his flower beds. While they were arguing his father arrived and took his brother's side. "My father called me a 'tin God.' My mother was very excited when she heard us quarreling, but she said nothing. For the first time I talked back to my father. I told him that he had no right making cracks like that 'tin God' stuff at me. He was so angry I could swear that he was going to hit me. I was scared deep inside, but I enjoyed the fight, particularly at the moment when my mother came in. I was also happy to tell my brother off. When I noticed that my mother was watching I gave them hell. I did not care what they had to say."

Doctor: You emphasize your satisfaction particularly when your mother was watching. Did you feel this way at that time, or are you feeling this way while you are recounting all this to me just now?

Patient: No, I felt this way at the time. It was so much fun to see my father get so infuriated. He didn't even make sense. He mumbled along. It was at that point that my mother intervened. She asked us all to be quiet and said it was silly to argue like children. She was angry. At that moment my resistance collapsed. I thought, "My father won't protect me this time"; and the thought crossed my mind, "Gee, how cruel the world is to me."

Doctor: Why blame the world? It was you who enjoyed the fight, and now you present yourself as the victim when your mother did not take your side.

Patient: My father was so angry that he didn't speak to me this morning. I had the feeling that he was jealous. My brother and my father seem always to be together. They seem to get along well and are always in competition with me. I have to avoid them.

Doctor: Yet you were the instigator of the fight, and now you are running away.

Patient (quite annoyed): I heard you before. I agree that it is true what you say, but I know that my mother prefers me.

The therapist here decides to confront the patient with his paradoxical feelings and emphasizes his becoming the victim while he enjoyed the fight. This clearly is annoying to the patient, but he is able to accept it and look at it.

Doctor: It seems to me that your relation with your mother is a much bigger problem in your life than your homosexual feelings which brought you to our clinic.

Patient: How could you say such a thing! You're supposed to help me, not to make me feel guilty. I feel mad at you, and I don't give a hoot about what you think.

The anxiety-provoking aspect of the therapist's confrontation is clear, but some reaction should be anticipated sooner or later.

Doctor: Yes, I know, in the same way you feel angry at your father.

He also draws a parallel between the patient's transference feelings for him and his feelings for his father.

Patient: Hell, yes; hell, no — I mean — I — I don't know what I'm saying. I feel mad at you, this is what I know, and I don't care what you think.

He continued like this for a while, and then he switched and started to describe his angry feelings toward his father, but toward the end of the hour he agreed that his relationship with his mother was a big problem to him.

He came ten minutes late for the next interview. He entered the office smiling broadly and announced that everything was much better at home. He also mentioned that during the week he had felt sad, had vague fears about being "incurable," and had thought of himself as a "hopeless case." All during the week he was angry at his professors and he did not study very well. "Hell, I don't give a hoot about my professors and what they think," he said.

Doctor: You seem to describe your feelings for the professors in the same language that you used for me as well as for your father last time.

Again the therapist chooses here to deal with the transference feelings rather than pursue the patient's associations to the "incurable hopeless" reactions.

Patient: You all meddle in my affair. I mean my affairs (blushing).

Doctor: With your mother!

Patient: I got mad at you last time, but you were right. During all this week I thought that it would be very nice to run away with my mother as my mistress. What a terrible thought! Yet it was at times like this that I felt very happy, elated, on top of the world.

Doctor: For an "incurable hopeless" case you seem to be doing pretty well! You can tell me about it; I understand.

Since the transference issues are very much alive the therapist decides to continue to deal with them; he also tends to minimize the importance of the patient's passive reactions.

Patient: When I was in the third grade I had a crush on my teacher. She was the best in the world. Once she gave me a thrashing for not preparing my lesson, and I felt completely dejected — like my mother pushing me off her lap.

He described the episode at length and said he had wished that the teacher would take his mother's place after his mother pushed him off her lap but, unfortunately, the teacher acted like his mother. "All women let you down"!

Doctor: And how do you feel then?

Patient: I feel cold inside. I look to my father for reassurance. I am a coward. There is all this tension and frightening feeling inside. It is as if he knows my secret. I feel guilty.

Doctor: What is this secret of yours all about? Have you committed some kind of offense?

Patient: Well, yes. All these thoughts that I have — all these things that I read in those sex magazines — the image of my mother always comes to mind. It is during those times that I think nobody cares about me. She doesn't care about me, the teacher doesn't care about me — no one gives a damn. I feel sorry for myself.

Doctor: There we go again. You feel sorry for yourself! This will not get you anywhere. It will not solve your conflict and your antagonism for your father. Don't forget, however, that if you look on your father for reassurance you must be fond of him. After all, we know how nice he had been to you in the past.

Patient: It is because of that that I feel guilty.

Doctor: Okay. Now what comes to mind?

Patient: When I feel this way I have no courage, as I told you. It is because I am a coward, and this is why I seek reassurance.

Doctor: Courage is to know that one feels like a coward at times and, despite this, to be able to decide and to act. All of us are afraid at times.

Patient: I know what you mean, Doctor. I don't feel like that all the time.

During the following interview the patient said that ever since the weekend fight with his father they had been getting along much better.

Doctor: I'm struck that you have not talked about your sister at all.

This is a mistake on the part of the therapist. It is clear from what follows that the patient's feelings for men are still a hot issue.

Patient: That's true. She's younger and married. I always felt a great deal of fondness for her. There was no real trouble between us, no real competition. It's my brother whom I dislike. You see, my sister was married young. I didn't like the guy she married, at first, but then I got used to him. However, she has gone away now, and it's quite some time — over a year. She lives in California. I feel my parents favor my brother. I am jealous and angry, and I want to kick him. Once I did. I knocked him out (blushing). I want to knock him out of my sight for good, once and for all. I have the same thought about my father. I wish to get rid of him. Do you understand — get rid of him. I want to be the boss.

Doctor: What about all this? You are not very guilty today.

Patient (as if awakening): It's tough, but I want to be the center of attention. Sex is the first thing that comes to my mind and in it the thought of sexual intercourse with women. Yet I don't get aroused . . .

Doctor (after a long pause): What are you thinking about?

Patient: . . . something, that is hard to talk about.

Doctor: Just what comes to mind?

Patient: It's the image of my mother, but there is something to do with women in general. The notion of sexual intercourse with a girl is not satisfying to me. There is something frightening, disgusting about it. For instance, I saw a woman on the subway. I was suddenly aroused. I had an erection. But suddenly that funny hurt feeling came all over me. I was no more aroused. The thought occurred to me, "I couldn't touch her," and you know what the reason would be? (Another pause.) It's because of last night. I was alone in the house with my mother. I had this strange feeling all over again. I didn't feel right. I didn't feel at ease. I have noticed this before, but I never realized that it was connected with my mother. You brought it into my mind.

Doctor: I did not. It was you who talked about it in a roundabout way. I tied it all together for you.

The rest of the time was spent in recapitulating what had already been learned in psychotherapy.

When he came for the next appointment the patient asked whether it would be possible for the clinic to accept a cash payment because he did not want the bill mailed to his house.

Doctor: Why not?

Patient: I want to evade the whole issue of psychiatry with my parents. I like to keep my parents guessing. It gives me satisfaction. I like to tell them big stories. I like to keep secrets. For instance, I enjoy teasing my mother. I suspect that sometimes maybe she is also thinking that something is going on between us. It's a terrible thing to think about, I know. My mother is forbidden to me. I now understand why I like so much to walk with only my underclothes on. My father always gets mad and tells me to get the hell out and put some clothes on. But my mother laughs and laughs. She gets a kick out of it, and my father gets so angry about it.

Doctor: Your father gets angry when you are exhibitionistic, and your mother enjoys it all. So you have your cake and eat it, too!

Patient: What do you mean? My father knows that I don't like girls.

Doctor: Exactly. So you play a "game" of being the homosexual to fool your father, while all the time you have your sexual thoughts about your mother. The thought that you're a homosexual makes you feel safe from your father's anger. How can he be angry at a homosexual! So you go on and have all the sexual wishes and images that you like. You have found a nice way to carry on your "affair" with your mother! It's a neurotic way!

Patient: This is all nonsense! Do you hear, *all* nonsense.

Doctor: You don't like to hear the truth.

Patient: I know you tried to help me, but this doesn't help me. It makes me mad.

Doctor: Because I know your secret?

Patient: If my father knew he'd kill me.

Doctor: Well, I'm not going to kill you. What is important is to be honest with yourself. Now what about the question of not sending the bill to your house?

Patient (hesitantly): I still wish you wouldn't. You know what people think about psychiatry?

Doctor: I don't care what other people think. I am interested only in what *you* think.

Patient: Well, you know psychiatry, head shrinkers, crazy stuff, and all that.

Doctor: So you think if the bill gets to your house your parents will think that you are "crazy and stuff like that"?

Patient: Yes, in a funny sort of way.

Doctor: In what way will being crazy upset you, since you know you are not?

Patient: Crazy people do crazy things.

Doctor: Such as?

Patient: Sexual and all that.

Doctor: So you are afraid that your father will become suspicious about your secret?

Patient: Yes, in a way.

Doctor: From what I know about you I know that you are tough; you are not some kind of weakling. You can take your own responsibility. Furthermore, I take psychiatry seriously, and I am not going to help you play destructive games. We are not going to send your bill anywhere else but to your own house. After we talked about courage last week you come and

ask me to go along and encourage your cowardly ways of
dealing with this situation. Now once and for all, I assume
that you are still interested in understanding yourself and not
in playing games.

Patient (pause): Okay, send it to my house and let all hell
break loose!

In the next interview he came in beaming. He announced
that he had no urge to masturbate and no fantasies of admiring men; but, what pleased him most was that he took a girl
out on a date after going to a football game. "We had fun
the whole afternoon and then we went out for dinner and
then to a show. Later on I sat in the back of the car and I took
Peg in my arms. I had three drinks and felt on top of the
world! I had a friendly feeling for her. I was happy about her.
Afterwards I felt mixed up. I felt I could have done much
more, but I didn't dare to try. I don't feel ready yet. And I
started thinking 'maybe it would do more harm than good.'
Throughout that time I kept on saying to myself, 'She's a
girl — she's a girl — not a fellow'! Well, it's kind of hard to
talk about all this. I don't want to tell you. It embarrasses me.

Doctor: You seem proud of it.

Patient: Of course I am.

Doctor: Now what about it?

Patient: It's none of your goddam business (blushing).

Doctor: It seems to me that you're doing with me what
you're doing with your father. You want to have a secret and
keep it to yourself.

Patient: I've never thought of it that way. I get angry at
your questions. Anyway, I plan to go to another football
game this week. (Pause.) I did a terrible thing. I lied to my
mother. I did not tell her that I was going to go out with
Peg. I said that I was going out with the fellows.

Doctor: Hmm.

Patient: I thought that my mother would be upset if I am
committed to someone else. It would hurt her. Peg is a good-
looking girl all around.

Doctor: There is no evidence of this. It is your wish that she
feels hurt.

Patient: Well, maybe. (Pause.) Oh, damn you. Yes, I know.

I want her to be jealous. As I told you, Peg is a good-looking girl. I like to talk to her, to do things to her. Maybe next time I'll try. Her boss likes her, too. He is a pain in the neck.

Doctor: Oh, oh!

Patient: I am telling you, he is a pain in the neck. He gets along so well with girls. It irritates me to see him — the way he talks to all these women — the way they look at him — they all drool. He is a good-looking, tall guy — grey hair, smart clothes, and all that.

He continued to talk about his jealous feelings for her boss.

He was again ten minutes late for the next interview. "It bothered me when I said that I did not want to tell you everything," he said, as he settled himself into the chair.

Doctor: Is that what bothered you, or that I said your feelings for me were similar to your feelings for your father?

He was silent and seemed to be in deep thought before he spoke.

Patient: I had a nasty dream. I had just finished talking to you in the interview. There was a great deal of commotion outside. You went out to see what it was all about. It was my mother outside, with a low-cut dress, her shoulders exposed. You could almost see her breasts. It was a beautiful red dress. You spoke to her. You both went away. I was furious at you, so I came running after you down the elevator, but my mother turned around to me and gave me hell for spending seventy-five dollars per session, but I smiled and I said, "The clinic is charging me only five dollars." That was the end of the dream.

Doctor: What associations come to mind about it?

Patient: My mother was so young in the dream — the low neckline. It was my mother at her best.

Doctor: What about your mother at her best?

Patient: I was furious. She belongs to someone else.

Doctor: What do you mean?

Patient: She is *my* mother.

Doctor: You mean she talks to me, she goes along with me in the elevator, and she leaves you.

Patient (angrily): You have no business with my mother. You're older and you take her away. Damn it.

Doctor: Let me remind you that this is *your dream.* Furthermore, your mother belongs to someone else, indeed.

Patient: Yes, and it makes me mad.

Doctor: But you have Peg.

Patient (smiling): Yes, thank goodness!

Doctor: Now what about the seventy-five dollars?

Patient: Well, seventy-five dollars is all that I have in my bank account. I don't know.

Doctor: So your mother thought in the dream that you should not spend all your money on psychiatry.

Patient: But I said it costs only five dollars.

Doctor: Does it mean that you have enough money for fifteen more sessions?

Patient: In a way, yes, because I think I can do the work we have to accomplish here in that time span.

Doctor: Yet you were angry with me in the dream for taking your mother away from you.

Patient: Yes, you see in the dream my mother does not want me to come to see you while she goes away with you. On the other hand, I say I want to see you for fifteen more times.

Doctor: The question is whether you want to see me fifteen more times so as to be with your mother and me, or is it because you want to make me abandon your mother to come back with you and continue psychotherapy?

Patient: Oh, no. I want you to abandon my mother and come back and give me psychotherapy. It is that I want my mother for myself.

Doctor: I know that, but then why not do what she wants you to do — to save your money?

Patient: I *want* her to be with me, not with you; but I also want to have psychotherapy with you because I like what we are doing here. I make progress here.

Doctor: It is having your cake and eating it too. Of course, it is a dream. In reality you have Peg.

Patient: Yes, this pleases me, and this is why I like our work. It is evident here that although this dream may not have been analyzed completely, it did in a limited way add to the overall understanding of the basic emotional conflict under-lying the patient's problem, which was defined originally and is in the process of being solved during psychotherapy. In this way dreams can be used advantageously in short-term anxiety-provoking psychotherapy.

Patient: I have the feeling that there is a part of me that can laugh at myself — at all these crazy things I'm thinking about, but there is another part which is full of all these desires. For the last two weeks I have had no sexual feelings for men and no "images." There were two or three girls at work I felt a sexual attraction for, but I resisted. I saw Peg. I was all excited but, as you know, I can't tell you everything.

Doctor: There we go again!

Patient: I hate to tell you. I did masturbate three times. Peg's image was in my mind (pause, seeming to hem and haw). Damn it — this is my own private business. (Then smiling:) Well, it's funny. I tried to get an image of the boy I used to think about when I masturbated, but I couldn't do it any more. Then Peg came to my mind all of a sudden. I had a terrific desire for her.

Doctor: I think the most difficult part in all this is for you to talk to me about it because I remind you of your father.

Patient: This is true. Particularly when I have these sexual thoughts in my mind and when you ask me these unpleasant questions.

Doctor: I know how you feel, but these are things which you must understand for yourself. This takes courage. We are here together to try to solve these problems which have bothered you for so long. I am here to help you, but I am not here to pat you on the back. My job is to ask you these unpleasant questions, so that you can do the job.

Patient: I know, Doctor, and I appreciate it. I like so much to see Peg again, but I'm worried. When I have to do things in reality I am afraid to get entangled.

It is significant that the patient, despite his angry feelings for his therapist, is able to work hard at trying to understand his problem.

In the following interview he again reiterated his loss of interest in boys. Then smiling, he added, "Maybe homosexuality is inside, hidden somewhere."

Doctor: It is possible. What do you think?

Patient: I am not interested in men. I look at them, and they leave me cold.

He seemed to be withdrawn, however. "Aren't you satisfied"? he asked.

Doctor: How are you feeling right now?

Patient: All of a sudden I feel terribly tired. I don't know what to say. I am off the track.

Doctor: Does it have to do with me?

Here, again, the therapist invites the patient to talk about his transference feelings, realizing full well that this will make the patient angry.

Patient (very angry): Why do you always bring this thing up! I feel very jealous. Any man is my enemy, now that I have these new interests in girls, but I don't know what to do about it. It's all so new, and I am so inexperienced. I hate bosses. I hate everybody, and you're the boss of this office. I object to your asking me questions about my women. What do you have to come into my business for? I am ready to tell you off. This morning I told off my boss. I wanted to get rid of him, but then suddenly I had the fear afterwards that he may not want to protect me any more, or even that he may want to get rid of me. It's like my dad. I have this feeling that he wants to reject me, to get rid of me, and not to protect me.

Doctor: But I thought you wanted to get rid of your boss?

Patient: Well, yes, that is true. I suppose it goes on something like this. If there were girls and I was interested in them I would be wronging the only one, my only one, so maybe it's better not to have any feelings at all.

Doctor: Who is that?

Patient: My mother, of course.

Doctor: What about Peg?

Patient: It's my relationship with Peg that's the big problem. What good does it do?

Doctor: Now, why are you tired?

Patient: Well, I had some fear before coming into the office, and it was then that I felt very tired.

He was silent for a while and then a broad smile appeared on his face. "I know what it is," he exclaimed triumphantly. He paused for a while and then he said, "When that girl came out of your office I thought I had seen her before. I only wanted to know who she was, but I was afraid to ask. I was just curious"!

Doctor: Just curious?

Patient: I just wanted to know who she was.

Doctor: Only?

Patient: Well, it's not the truth.

Doctor: Hmm?

Patient (silent for a while): Well, it isn't — it isn't that, uh (turning crimson) you know — (pause) well, uh, I was attracted to her . . . Are you going to kick me out?

Doctor: Okay, you know it, I know it, so let's look at what's going on in here, what your feelings are about all this, instead of all this hemming and hawing. These thoughts and emotions that you have about my female patient and myself seem to be similar to the feelings you have for your boss and the girls, and for your father and your mother. It seems you are curious about her, but you are afraid that I might retaliate. Thus, you felt weak as a way out. You feigned weakness with your father in the same way. You wanted my protection after your curiosity about my female patient in the same way as you wanted your father to protect you when you were interested in your mother. You use your weakness and your homo-sexuality as a kind of excuse not to go out with girls, so as not to be unfaithful to your mother, as well as to fool your father. Killing two birds with one stone.

The rest of the hour was spent essentially on giving examples of the patterns of this behavior. Toward the end of the hour the patient smiled with a sigh of relief.

The next time he again brought in a dream. There was a girl whom he was kissing. She was wearing a beautiful dress which belonged to his mother. He said that he was feeling much better after our last hour. He had the impression that things were clearing up.

Doctor: Well, tell me about it.

Patient: When I was able to say exactly what I had in my own mind last time about feeling weak, and when you pointed out what happened, I felt good. After I left here I had a wonderful week. I seem to be noticing that this world is full of pretty girls! At times I think how foolish it all is for me to keep my interest all locked inside. I have wasted so much precious time. I realize that you have encouraged me to keep my interests up in order to get freer. I realize that all men don't have the opportunity that I have in my job. I am surrounded by beautiful women! Yet, two days ago I regressed a little bit. I saw a young man and I had some feelings for him, but I know why it happened. It was after I had talked to my mother about sex, and my mother said that I must mix more with girls. She even suggested places where I might be able to go and meet them. She said, "You must have many girls." I suddenly felt queer inside me, inside the pit of my stomach, and felt that my hands were shaking. The thought crossed my mind — she's pushing me away. I don't want to be pushed. I don't want my brother and my father to hear my conversation. I want my mother to myself. You see, she was pleased to talk to me and told me that she dated a lot before getting married. She had a lot of boy friends. When she said what she did I felt sore at her. I wanted to grab her. I wanted to hurt her.

Doctor: Grab her? Or hurt her?

Patient: Both. You know what I mean. She was wearing that beautiful dress, yet she was pushing me away. From then on I felt cold inside for the rest of the night. It was that night that I had a dream about slapping my mother.

Doctor: You didn't tell me about that dream.

Patient: That was all there was to it. When I woke up I was irritated at my brother, who was making a lot of noise. My father seemed to pay no attention to me. No one cared. I went to work. It was there that I saw this guy. He really didn't appeal to me. The thought just crossed my mind — I'll tell my mother I like men to punish her, so that she won't push me away and try to make me go out with girls.

Doctor: What about women's dresses? You know, we still don't understand that clearly. Now the girl in the dream wears your mother's dress.

Patient: Yes.

Doctor: And she is very attractive?

Patient: Yes.

Doctor: Sexually?

Patient: Yes.

Doctor: Well, it is interesting, because the image you had when masturbating, about that boy who is built like a girl, and was wearing —

Patient (interrupting): Oh, my God — Oh, no!

Doctor: Yes.

Patient: I never thought of it this way all this time. You read about all that stuff in magazines; but sex with my mother in that way! It is horrible!

Doctor: Not really. After all, even in your dream you had to camouflage the situation. Don't forget she was a boy with no face. He just wore your mother's dress!

After this stormy session one may anticipate a reaction during the next hour.

In the next interview the patient said that he had almost forgotten about his psychotherapy hour. He had a wish to get away from it all, to quit school and go somewhere, maybe to Alaska during the summer to climb mountains. Away from women. "I feel I am being pushed around."

Doctor: What are you running away from?

Patient: Well, the other day after a date with Peg I felt very excited. She gave me her picture. She looked cute. I kept on looking at the picture, and then I masturbated. I was never more satisfied in my whole life. You know, Doctor, I actually enjoy being pushed around.

Doctor: I know you do.

Patient: You do some of the work for a while, and I'll relax.

Doctor: This is not what you're here for.

The therapist here avoids getting entangled into passive wishes of the patient.

He paused and looked angry. Staring at my dictating machine, he said, "Are you recording what I said? Who is doing the typing? After all, it's nobody's business but my own." Then, smiling, he continued, "I have noticed it in the last few sessions, but I realize that this is silly business. You see, I have a feeling that I've learned a great deal in my sessions with you. In some kind of a way I want to think of you as a friend of mine. In many ways this is the way I feel about my father. I suppose I get into fights with my father as I get into fights with you, but when my father is nice to me he is a friend. I have the feeling that you're not a friend of mine because I pay the clinic to see you. A thought just crossed my mind that you remind me of Bob. Bob is a good kid. He is a friend of mine. We had much fun together last summer; but recently I thought that Bob might take Peg away from me, and then suddenly I felt mad at Bob. I wanted to tear him apart — to give him hell. It was then that I talked about your dictating machine."

Doctor: Isn't there something else about my dictating machine?

Patient: No, that's all.

Doctor: You said something about someone typing.

Patient (sheepishly): Well, I had a thought that maybe . . .

Doctor: You mean the person who types my notes.

Patient: Yes, she may be interested in what I have to say . . . You remember I want to be the center of attention.

Doctor: Yes, I know only too well!

The next week he was jubilant. He had had three dates with Peg and described all this in detail. Finally, they were thinking of "going steady." He was able to talk to his mother about Peg. "She seemed, of all things, to like the idea. She did not appear to be disappointed as I had expected her to be."

Doctor: As I am sure you know by now, it is your expectations and your wishes rather than what is happening in reality that make you see things the way you want to.

In the next two sessions he spent most of the time on his detailed descriptions of his dates with Peg and on the fun they had together. Toward the end of the session, he said, "It seems to me that things have been very different during the last four weeks. I am feeling better and, although I expect the fear of homosexuality may return, it does not bother me so much to think about it. Something unusual seems to have happened. You have helped me learn to look into problems and to realize that they are within me and are not someone else's. I have a way now to understand myself. Things are getting along with Peg. I was thinking that I get along with my dad much better. Do you think that I may be able to carry on without your help from now on"?

Doctor: What do you think?

Patient: I think so.

Doctor: I'm in agreement. You have made a great deal of progress and seem to understand some of your wishes and your fears. We have traced your feelings to your attachment to your mother; we understand your competition and anger with your father, as you expressed repeatedly to me, particularly lately. Furthermore, we know you like your father. This work here seems to have helped your relationship with your father to improve. You have been able to see your mother more realistically and find a substitute in Peg for your sexual feelings for her. You don't have to pretend to be a homosexual any more. Yes, I agree we should stop psychotherapy after two more sessions.

The last two sessions were spent essentially in the patient's narration of his happy times with Peg. He also talked with some vague apprehension about termination, and this issue was dealt with explicitly. During the last interview he mentioned that he continued to get along quite well with his father and brother. "I can't understand it. My father and brother seem to be different people."

Doctor: They have not changed. You are the one who has.

Patient: I get along with them. We don't seem to have much to fight about these days.

Doctor: Of course, you don't. You used to have quarrels when you had a problem. Now you have solved it.

The patient smiled broadly.

A follow-up interview in a year's time was agreed upon, and therapy was terminated. In follow-up he said that he was feeling fine. He told us that after the end of psychotherapy he became engaged to Peg. The engagement had lasted for about six months, during which time he realized that there were many serious differences between the two of them. They broke off the engagement. He went out very frequently after this on dates. Finally he was married. He said that he had put into use the things he had learned about himself in psychotherapy. He felt fine, and was proud to be "his own boss." His homosexual fears had disappeared.

Discussion

Homosexuality presents the therapist with a dilemma. Is it used defensively to cover up the patient's incestuous heterosexual wishes, or is it a more basic way of life which gives rise to difficulties? The first possibility is amenable to change as a result of short-term anxiety-provoking psychotherapy. The patient usually wants to get rid of his homosexual tendencies. In the second instance the patient is unwilling to alter his homosexual ways. What he does want is to eliminate the unpleasant emotions which arise as a result of conflicts between his homosexual desires and the attitudes of society.

The patient was clearly motivated to change outwardly, but as one witnessed in the course of his therapy, he was unwilling to give up the advantages which his pseudohomosexuality offered to him by keeping him attached to his mother and detached from his unsuspecting father. The transference relationship was stormy despite his tendency at times to become passive and to feign weakness. His motivation to stand on his own two feet and to understand his problems was strong. It was as a result of this perseverance that he was able to succeed. It may be of interest to notice that the therapist was able to gauge his patient's progress in psychotherapy by observing the development of his relationship with Peg, and how he was able to interpret the patient's dream about the girl who wore his mother's dress to help bring to consciousness his powerful incestuous desires for her. The follow-up points to the complete resolution of the patient's emotional conflicts and the disappearance of his homosexuality.

11

ANXIETY AND EXAMINATION PHOBIA

A seventeen-year-old college freshman came to the psychiatry clinic because of an onset of acute anxiety four weeks before final examinations. She said that since September of the previous year she had experienced apprehension at the time of various quizzes or when she was pressed to hand in a paper on time. She described her difficulties as follows: "My anxiety increases as soon as I know that I have to write a paper. I feel a sense of pressure which increases until it becomes almost unbearable. All kinds of terrible thoughts flood my head. I think that I will never be able to finish it on time, and soon after, I usually become frantic and I rush around trying to explain to various people, such as my roommate, the secretary of the department, or my instructor, that there is no conceivable possibility for me to hand in my paper on time." She emphasized, however, that she seriously doubted her ability to continue to do this in the future. She described how, on the occasion when she actually was one week late in handing in one of her papers, she was surprised that the instructor had smiled and appeared to be very understanding about it all. Once she was able to get a postponement, but she felt guilty about "winning," and was preoccupied with the idea that she had manipulated the "innocent" instructor to give her an extra week. She also had the fantasy that the chairman of the department would be very angry with him and that he could conceivably lose his job. Despite this, she asked for a second one-day postponement.

Procrastinations about when to start or how to begin to write took a great deal of her valuable time. She described all this as "torture" or "agony." Her papers were always excellent, but she was never satisfied with them. The same difficulties occurred before hour examinations. Having to prepare herself for a quiz was invariably associated with tension and was followed by the thought that she would become paralyzed and unable to function altogether; yet, despite all these feelings, she was able to take the midyear examinations, to think that she had flunked, and to discover, to her surprise, that she got straight A's. These grades, however, did not influence her subsequent behavior about papers and examinations, and her compulsion to convince everybody that she needed postponements, that she had to be handled in a special way, or that everybody was very nice to her because, realistically, she was not worth the grade which she had received, continued. The thought that one day her inadequacy was going to be "discovered" and then she would "flunk out" and have to leave college was a constant presence in the back of her mind.

Four weeks before her final exams she became acutely panicky after she heard that one of the girls had decided to be married and give up college. She described this as follows: "I was talking with my roommate when Jane burst into the room, looking flushed, beamed, and said that her parents did not object to her plan to marry Bill, even though it meant that she would have to leave college. My roommate screamed and kissed Jane, and they both started to cry. I was thunderstruck! What foolishness, I thought, what goings on, what a sophomoric behavior! I tried to smile, but I couldn't. I just muttered, 'I am glad for you, Jane, but in the long run education is very important.' I somehow wanted to say something else, to add something nice, but I couldn't. Education *is* very important. This I had heard all my life from my mother, and I was convinced it was correct. I thought of all the torture I was going through about education, and there was Jane, without batting an eye, giving up the best women's college in America. What a fool, I thought, yet deep inside I felt perplexed — almost awed by her courage to do what she did." Then she added, "Of course, all this must sound ridiculous to you." And then, after a pause, "Do you follow what I am trying to tell you"?

The next day she was acutely uncomfortable because she was absolutely convinced that she was going to fail her finals, that a great catastrophe would befall her, and finally that she would have to leave the college in disgrace. She was able to talk to her roommate, who knew about the psychiatry clinic, but she delayed calling for an appointment. It was the announcement of the engagement of yet another girl that precipitated her coming to the clinic for help.

The patient was a tall, thin, bony person, with stringy blonde hair. She was plainly dressed in an old sweater, an unmatching skirt, and old loafers. She was born in France, but her parents had emigrated to the United States in 1951, when she was ten years old. She spoke several languages very well.

She described her mother as a "brilliant woman" who had graduated from the Sorbonne. She considered her to be a "superior human being" and was very close to her. Her mother, in turn, was proud of her daughter, and the two of them viewed themselves as being above the rest of the family, which consisted of her father and two brothers. Her mother was also described as making all the important decisions, particularly in financial matters, such as the family investments. In addition, several relatives also sought her financial advice.

Her father was three years younger than her mother. He was a lawyer, a graduate of the Paris Law School, but he was looked down upon by his wife, despite the fact that he was very successful financially, particularly after the family came to the United States. The patient had two younger brothers with whom she did not get along. They were both close to their father. One of her brothers was a good athlete in high school, but the patient wondered whether he would have "the intelligence to go to college" because his grades were not very good.

She described her early life in Europe, remembering many details about several ski trips the whole family took together. Talking about her mother she said, "Living close to a genius is the most satisfying experience, better than all the mediocre company that one may have in a lifetime." She gave this as an excuse for not getting along with other children in school, feeling superior to all of them, even including some of the teachers. Her academic performance was, nevertheless, outstanding; yet she was, even at that time, apprehensive about her grades. She claimed that France was "the only civilized country in the world." She liked English literature, however, and there were several American writers that she admired. She proceeded as if giving a lecture. "You know that Poe is great, but he is not appreciated here as he should be. There are a few others, too, like Lewis and O'Neill. Everybody is preoccupied with money in this country. Materialism reigns supreme, nobody reads — not even the newspapers, or, if they do, they start with the funnies or the sports pages. There is a naive admiration of Americans for France. Everything French is fashionable, from clothes, perfumes, and champagne to such foolishness as french kissing." At this point she blushed and changed the subject.

She was accepted at several colleges, and, after a great deal of discussion with her mother, they both agreed that she must go to the "best college," where, of course, she was admitted. Her relations with men were few and far between. She went out on a few dates during high school, and although she looked down on boys, she talked with warmth about two of her cousins to whom she was very attached; but she added quickly that the reason for this was that she considered them to be of superior intellect. She said that they used to play together and added that she loved to share her own lunch with them because they liked the delicacies which her mother always prepared for her and put into her lunch box. She was also very close to her maternal grandfather, who was also described as brilliant but totally uneducated.

When asked about what she expected from psychotherapy, she answered that she was dissatisfied with all this fear of examinations, which, although it had become acute lately, had been present for a long time. She said that she felt sure she had the ability to understand intellectually the reasons for her difficulties, but she was aware that fears and anxieties were emotions. She then went on to say: "As you probably know, the French always pride themselves on their rational way of looking on life; but, in the emotional area they are just as vulnerable as anyone else. This weakness, I am afraid, is also part of me, thus I need guidance to help me disentangle my problem. I am sure that I can do the job." She smiled and added, "There is a general feeling of dissatisfaction about my life and my relations with men."

The patient's brilliance was obvious. It was thought during the evaluation that, despite her apparent conviction of feminine superiority, she did relate well with the interviewer and was able to show emotion during the interview when she talked about her mother, her cousins, and her grandfather. She seemed to be motivated to understand the reasons for her symptoms and to realize that she had to work hard. When asked what sacrifices she was prepared to make, she answered that she was willing to cut some of her classes in order to keep her appointments in the clinic, despite the difficulties this might create for her. She asked to pay the clinic fee, which she could afford, out of her own allowance. "After all," she said, "this is *my* psychotherapy."

The diagnosis of psychoneurosis with obsessive and phobic features was made, and short-term anxiety-provoking psychotherapy was suggested to the patient. She eagerly accepted our offer.

In her second interview she appeared cold and distant and asked for a change in the appointment time because this created a conflict with one of her courses. The therapist was quiet, and she went on to describe her feelings about the fear of examinations, without waiting for an answer. Most of the interview was spent on history-taking, which was not very different from what had been obtained in the evaluation interview. Toward the end of the hour the patient described her fear as follows: "What usually happens is that I decide to go to the library in order to do some studying, but once there

I find so many fascinating books, full of interesting things to read, that I get distracted. What I find myself doing is opening a book, leafing right through it, and the next thing I know is that I have read a hundred pages and have spent two hours, which I should have used for studying. Valuable time is lost, and I start getting nervous. In this way I don't prepare myself adequately for my exams or for my papers. By the end of the day I have collected a lot of interesting information, but it all amounts to having done no work. Since I always expect to write a "perfect" paper, I start feeling more anxious and so it goes."

Doctor: Can you describe these anxious feelings for me?

Patient: (After being silent for a while, she snapped irritably): You know what anxiety is, don't you? It is not different with me than it is with anyone else!

Doctor: This may be so, but I am interested in your anxiety, not in anyone else's.

Patient: Well . . . I feel a need to talk to my friends about this, but I haven't discussed it with anybody. (Pause.) Come to think of it, this is not true. I did discuss it with my room-mate, but she is an unusually intelligent girl. She is not as bright as I am, however.

Doctor: Have you discussed it with anyone else?

Patient: No, I have not. On one occasion I remember I had the thought that I might, but I haven't. It was when these anxious feelings started to bother me a great deal I thought I should speak to my brother. This is peculiar . . . inconceivable in fact. I changed my mind because he was a man. You see, I don't talk about my emotional feelings with my father.

Doctor: But you are here to discuss your emotional feelings, aren't you?

Patient: Oh, well, this is different. (She blushed.) It *is* different.

Doctor: Yes. Now what about this anxious feeling. What comes to mind?

Patient: It is associated with my mother, and this worries me.

Doctor: Why with your mother?

Patient: Because I am absolutely sure that if I flunk my exam this would be a catastrophic blow to my mother. You see, my mother's life really depends on my doing well. After all, as you know, she always has emphasized her intellectual superiority over my father. Yet my father is an excellent lawyer and is making a great deal of money, and this is important in this country. My mother used my father. She claimed that he never gave her any intellectual stimulation and always had some kind of derogatory remarks to make about him. All this is in the record, anway, and I assume you must have read it, haven't you?

Doctor: You seem to show the same derogatory attitude to me as you describe your mother has for your father.

Since transference issues have come up so early in therapy it was decided that the patient should be confronted with them.

Patient (blushing): . . . It is true in a way. I do think that women are superior to men.

Doctor: You seem to have emphasized this point repeatedly, yet you also said that your father is successful. What do you make of this? After all, isn't this important too?

Patient: Yes, you see I can afford to see the most expensive psychiatrist. Can't you see that this is terribly important for me to get the money out of my own allowance?

Doctor: I'm not so sure about that.

Patient: This would be the only way that my mother would approve, if I paid for my own psychotherapy. My mother has had always some money of her own. It is she who pays for my college tuition. She feels that she must contribute for my education because, in her opinion, it is the most important thing that she can do for me.

Doctor: But if you flunk out it would mean that you disagree with her.

Patient: Yes. This is why I'm terrified. I don't disagree — I *agree* with my mother.

Doctor: Could it be that there is a part inside you that doesn't?

Patient (silent for a while): I can see your logic. (She was again silent for a while, and then:) Now what about the change of the hour?

Doctor: I understand that you have a conflict of interest, but my schedule is somewhat rigid, and this is the only hour I have.

One may view the therapist's attitude on this point as inflexible; but, in his judgment, he has to assess the patient's manipulative tendencies and her somewhat contemptuous attempt to make psychotherapy rank second to her studies. He, therefore, decides at this early point to draw the line.

Patient: I can understand that you cannot change, but will you please try to see if you can?

Doctor: Now first things first. It seems to me that before we discuss change in hours we must decide what problem you would like to solve in your treatment. From what I can see, it seems that these fears of examinations reflect your identification with your mother's views about education and feminine superiority, yet there is an element in all this that makes you apprehensive about accepting totally those views of your mother. Let me put it another way. You seem to have some doubts about accepting totally those views of your mother. You seem to have some doubts about accepting your mother's concept of femininity. If so, do you want to explore this area in psychotherapy, even if this means that you have to examine your relations and feelings with men, prosaic as they may be?

Patient: Well, I knew you were going to put it in this way, but I agree. Anyway, it is worth it, and if it proves the obvious . . . (She was silent for a while and then): Now what about the change of the time? Have you had time to think about it?

Doctor: What I said stands. If you want to see me it would have to be at this hour.

Patient: You are going to become the reason for my flunking my exam.

Doctor: Oh, come now, Miss N., I am surprised at you! After telling me that you are such a rational person and that you come from such a rational country, after emphasizing that you and your mother always think logically, after viewing me in a derogatory way, how could it be possible that *I* would be held responsible for *your* failing your exam?

At this point the patient turned crimson, not with anger, but with what appeared to be shame. It was almost as if she fell apart. For a while she sat looking at the floor without saying anything, and finally she muttered, "There is something in what you have said. I have felt it before, but somehow I cannot put it in words." We decided to meet at the same time the following week.

She came a few minutes late for the third interview and appeared again to be cold and distant. She apologized and said that there was a lot of traffic and that, as she had expected, it was difficult for her to make the interview on time. She added, almost imploring me, "Of course, it would be much more convenient for me if we changed the hour."

Doctor: You seem to have a different attitude about this subject today compared with the way you felt at the end of last week's interview. Are you aware of it?

Patient: Well, if you mean that I was a little flustered at what you said? Yes, it is true, but it seems inconsequential now. Could you possibly change this hour for me?

Doctor: No.

Patient: Well, I didn't expect you would. (Smiling warmly, she seemed satisfied at the answer and proceeded as follows:) I was unable to study at all during the week. My first final exam is in two days from today.

She then described how while attempting to study at the library she had found a copy of the Sunday *New York Times*, and had spent the afternoon reading and enjoying it. She mentioned that she always liked to read about international politics. She admitted that she resented the need to study for a "foolish exam." When the owner of the paper, a male student, asked her to return it to him, she felt very angry: "I was just reading about the autumn fashions, all about the new collections from Paris! I asked him if I could keep it for a while, but he apologized and said that it belonged to his girl friend from whom he had borrowed it and had to return it to her. Still feeling mad I blurted out, 'Next time why don't you borrow my copy of the *New York Times?*' "

Doctor: Your copy?

Patient: Yes, I don't know why I said this. After all, I did not have a copy.

Doctor: Maybe you wanted to have one so that you would lend it to the young man, rather than his borrowing it from another girl?

Smiling, she added, "You know, he was cute." She then associated to the good times with her two male cousins and said that she was always worried about what her father would think.

Doctor: Why your father?

Patient: Well, other women find my father very attractive. Of course, for people who are interested in things like that and have nothing more important to think about . . .

Doctor: You mean people like you.

Patient (blushing): What do you mean?

Doctor: You know what I mean — reading about the Parisian autumn fashions, male students, attractive men!

Patient: Well, you know, my brothers are also attractive. John, in particular, has several girl friends and gets along very well with them. I feel annoyed about all these foolish females who are running after boys. Screaming teenagers and all that nonsense. (She again switched to the subject of her worries and fears about her examinations and added that she could not conceive of the possibility that she would be able to pass at the rate that she was going.)

In the next interview she seemed very upset. She had taken three exams and had two more left. She was worried about these two and was convinced that she would fail.

Doctor: How did you do in the ones you took?

Patient (interrupting irritably): It's not the point. Can't you see that I am really worried about what is coming, not what has happened in the past?

Doctor: I am interested to know how you did in the ones you took.

Patient: This is not the point. Actually, I did not do so bad because I had done a little work; but what I am worried about is that I am convinced that I have no hope for the ones I have to take. I have done no work. I am totally unprepared.

The patient's irritation is understandable. In retrospect there was no reason why the therapist pursued the issue of the grades, because of his curiosity or his worry.

Doctor: Have you got your grades yet?

Patient: Yes.

Doctor: What were your grades for the exams that you have already taken?

Patient: They gave me good grades. But I am sure they have not looked carefully at my blue books. I am sure that I had not done so well. You see, they let the teaching fellows correct the exams. The professors have no time. They are too busy going to Washington or making speeches. If they did they would have flunked me. In the Sorbonne it is the professor who corrects the papers. Anyway, that is what they did in my mother's time. They are very much interested in the students. It is a superior educational system. The lectures are fascinating, always brilliant.

Doctor: This may be the case, but any student can buy the lecture series at any bookstore on the Boulevard St. Michel.

Finally the therapist returns to the task of doing anxiety-provoking psychotherapy.

Patient (with amazement): Oh, you know about the "cours polycopies." Well, yes, that part of it is not so good. I have also thought about it when my mother raved about the Sorbonne. This is also what my father had once said.

Doctor: Yet a minute ago you were parroting your mother in your exhortation of the superiority of the French system. Were you talking to me or to your father?

Patient: I had a queer feeling — the same thing that I experienced during the first hour — while you were talking, but I can't express it . . . Anyway, I didn't do so bad in those three courses.

Doctor: Isn't that good enough?

Again the therapist misses the point by this spontaneous remark.

Patient: Well, you see, I suspect they realized that I have an emotional problem in this area. By coming over here it means there is something wrong with me. That's why they gave me the good grades.

Doctor: So you use your emotional problem as a way for others to feel sorry for you.

Patient: I feel embarrassed. There is something like a vague threat about it all.

Doctor: Why do you have to cover up this apprehension of yours with this tough exterior? What does it feel like to be embarrassed?

Patient: It is like losing something precious, like losing my mind.

Doctor: What about that?

Patient: Losing the one thing my mother thinks is the most important thing in the world — my brains.

Doctor: What your mother thinks! . . . (not waiting for an answer) I think you exaggerate the importance of your brains to impress me, but I do not really think that you value your brains as much. I get the impression that you parrot your mother in order to hide something from her.

Patient: It's a funny feeling. My whole future seems to be at stake. (Smiling.)

Doctor: Why is it funny?

Patient: Well, "funny" is a matter of talking.

Doctor: But you use the word 'funny.' What is so funny about such a tragedy?

Patient: You see, on the one hand I feel that my whole future is at stake; at the same time there is something in me that enjoys the prospect of flunking, because, as you know, I have never flunked out in my whole life. Just even considering the idea gives me a perverse kind of a pleasure.

Doctor: What would happen in you flunked?

Patient: I would be more carefree; nothing would matter from then on. (She giggled at this point.)

Doctor: You mean to say you would be like those giggly teenagers who ran after your brother.

She looked a bit taken aback, but then she started to laugh and said, "I never thought you had it in you"!

Doctor: Please explain what you mean.

Patient: You seem to have understood something about me that I thought I was the only one who knew about.

Doctor: You mean to say that there is a part of you that is very feminine and likes boys.

Patient: The way you put it makes me mad. It isn't exactly like that . . .

Doctor (interrupting): It is exactly like that and you know it perfectly well.

Patient: But if . . .

Doctor: There are no ifs and buts. We know your feelings about your father and your cousins, the handsome student at the library, and this also includes me. You like men in a feminine way, but this gets you in trouble with the intellectual part of your personality — this so-called superior part, which comes from your identification with your mother. After all, your mother has a feminine side, too. Aren't you entitled to one, also?

Patient: What about my mother being feminine?

Doctor: Well, she did have three children, after all, didn't she?

The patient was silent for a long time and looked thoughtful. Then she said, "Sex was always a difficult subject for me. I remember when I was little, on my way back from school I followed a boy. I liked him, but I was so frightened that my mother would disapprove. As you can see, these feelings of mine are quite old." (She smiled.)

Doctor: Why did you smile?

Patient: The thought that crossed my mind was that is what psychiatric books are all about. I think you are right. I know what you mean, but it is so difficult to face all this.

She spent most of the following two hours talking about her intellectual superiority. An effort was made to get back to the subject of her femininity, but she seemed to be determined — almost having made up her mind on purpose — not to talk about her relations with men. Finally this resistance was pointed out to her.

Doctor: You are avoiding and have been avoiding talking about your feelings for men.

Patient: What do you mean?

Doctor: You know exactly what I mean. You said that it was difficult to face all this. I understand, but I do think that you must face these issues and not try to run away as you have been doing today and last week.

She came a half-hour early for her seventh interview and seemed to be more relaxed. She admitted that she had been thinking about the end of our previous interview the whole week long.

Patient: There is another thing that I remembered and I have never told anyone before. When I was fourteen I met a boy who was three years older. He was an avid skier, and on one occasion he asked me to go skiing with him, but I was terrified by the idea. I decided, finally, to accept his invitation, but I thought it would be better not to mention it to my mother. As a matter of fact, I lied to her. I told her that I was planning to stay overnight with a girl friend of mine to prepare for an exam. I don't remember whether my mother was suspicious or not. I suspect that she might have been. She didn't say a thing. So I went. We spent the night together. You know what he did? (She blushed.) He kissed me.

Doctor: He did, did he?

Patient (continuing to blush): You know what I mean. It was a great, warm feeling. (She had an ecstatic look on her face.)

It was pointed out to her that she had used the preparation for an examination as the very excuse to lie to her mother.

Doctor: Does, then, the fear of flunking an examination represent a wish which has to do with a strong desire for men?

She was silent and looked perplexed, but since it was at the end of the hour, it was left that she should think about it and we could discuss it the next time.

In the next interview she again came early and announced that she did not feel as intensely afraid about her exams any more. As usual she had passed all her exams with flying colors.

Patient: Somehow or other I don't think that they gave me special grades. It does not seem to be so important any more.

She described an episode which occurred in the library when a student helped her to carry some of her books. He said, "My, you are reading a lot these days," and I answered that I would rather be sailing on the Charles on a hot day like this. He looked at me and said, "I thought you hated the outdoors." I answered that it was a joke and that I really hated sailing.

Doctor: Why did you lie?

Patient (blushing): Well, you know, he may have asked me to go sailing with him, and you never know where these things end.

Doctor: Meaning?

Patient: If you start going out on dates and you get involved and pretty soon you are going steady, then . . .

Doctor: Oh! Is this the way it goes?

Patient: Stop being sarcastic!

Doctor: I did not mean to be sarcastic. It is the tone of your voice that amused me.

Patient: He is a nice kind of a fellow.

Doctor: He has no name?

Patient: Well . . . yes . . . His name is Don. By the way, there is one more thing that I never told anyone.

Doctor: Is this a confession, or do you think it is something of importance?

Patient: I don't mean it as a confession. It is just that it occurred to me, and I thought it was important to bring it up here to try to understand it.

Doctor: Fine. Go ahead.

Patient: When I was a little girl in France my father was telling me a story. We were sitting on the shore of the Lac du Bourget.

Doctor: "O lac . . . ils ont aimé!" Lamartine, eh?

Patient: Oh, stop it. I mean it. I was sitting on his lap. I had such a warm feeling. I must have been about five years old. I don't know exactly what happened, but somehow I was drenched when we went back home. My grandmother, my mother's mother, in whose house we were staying was very upset, and I remember having this scary feeling inside. Several years later, in New York, my mother and I were discussing poetry. There was quite a difference of opinion. I don't know what it was all about, but she was quite annoyed with me when I told her I liked Baudelaire. (She went on, in the same vein and imitating her mother's voice.) "I don't see how a girl like you could like such a sensuous poet, anyway, poetry is nonsense. It is for weak intellects. Now, philosophy is another matter — Bergson, for instance . . . " But as she went on I felt the same way. The same fear, yet I had the urge at the same time to go for a walk. I actually did, later on. It was a lovely day, and I went for a walk by the river.

Doctor: Hmm!

Patient: Yes, and I know what you mean. I had a sudden wish that I might get picked up by someone, but I thought it was absurd. At that moment I heard some voices, and I realized that there might be some men around there. I got terrified. It was absurd, I know, but one reads such reports in the newspapers.

Doctor: You mean the *New York Times?*

Patient (blushing): Yes, in a way.

Doctor: Now what about all this?

Patient: I was terrified, yet suddenly there was a feeling inside me that I would have liked something to happen.

Doctor: A warm feeling. (Turning crimson, she was silent.) Go on. Do you think that this wish of yours had something to do with the episode with your father when you were young?

She continued to be silent for a while.

Patient: I never thought of it. Well, no, it is not exactly the truth.

Doctor: It seems likely, since these two episodes are connected in your mind together. What do you think?

Patient: You know, honestly I have always looked down upon my father, but at times I know I exaggerated. I also tried to put on an act when I talked to you about him. But deep inside I know that there is a change more recently. In the past things were different. Maybe it was more so within the past four years. Maybe a little longer than that. I don't know. I guess it was . . . Well, as a child I was very fond of my father. Something happened, when I was about six or seven years old. I don't know what it was.

In the next two interviews the patient continued to talk about her childhood experiences. It became progressively clear that she had been very attached to her father when she was a child. It seems that her father left the family to come to the United States when the patient was six and a half years old, in order to arrange for the whole family to emigrate to this country. The patient remembered and recounted a dramatic scene when she was holding on to her father the day that he departed — sobbing and asking him not to leave, while her mother was pulling her away from him. She cried continuously, and that night she dreamed that her father was dead. The next day she felt fine. It was from then on that she dated the change in her feelings for her father. From then on also she started to look down on men. She became very close to her mother and began to admire her intellectual superiority. She was surprised that she had forgotten completely this episode about her father's departure, which seemed to have played such an important role in changing her attitude for him.

Doctor: I think that you were angry at your father for having abandoned you. It is also possible that you were jealous.

Patient: I don't know about that, but I can certainly trace my feelings of anger at him from then on.

In the next two interviews she talked about her childhood in France and very little about her anxiety for examinations and papers.

Doctor: Do you think that there is a change in you? I have not heard a word about exams recently. Of course you don't have to think about them until September.

She looked disinterested and brushed this question off in her usual fashion. "All this talk couldn't really contribute to any basic changes," she said. She was silent for a while, and then she smiled warmly.

Patient: Oh . . . I don't really mean it.

Doctor: You seem to smile. I suspect that you agree with

me. Intellect does not reign supreme any more! Being a woman has the upper hand!

In the thirteenth interview she announced that for the first time that she had had a dream. She was wandering along the shores of a beautiful river. She was a fairy. An old man with a cane was walking along a tortuous path. He seemed to be limping. She went to see if she could help, but suddenly he started to chase her, waving his cane at her. She woke up frightened.

Doctor: What are your associations to this dream?

Patient: Oh, it was some kind of a nightmare. I was quite anxious.

Doctor: What about the fairy?

Patient: You know, fairies are powerful. They can turn you into anything you want.

Doctor: So you are a powerful girl; but, interestingly enough, your magical powers have failed. You ended by being chased by the man.

Patient: I haven't thought of it this way. Actually — well, I don't know!

Doctor: What do you mean?

Patient: I had the feeling that something happened to him. He changed.

Doctor: He changed?

Patient: There was something about his changing.

Doctor: You mean by your own powers, as a fairy?

Patient (blushing): Something like that. He turned out to be much younger at the end.

Doctor: Anything else comes to mind about this dream?

Patient: I know what you mean. I thought you might be interested to hear about my dream. You psychiatrists like dreams, don't you?

Doctor: You mean to say that you brought it to me as a gift?

Patient: Yes, come to think of it, this man in the dream looked very much like you.

Doctor: Thank you, but you know, I do think that you have changed!

From then on the psychotherapy proceeded uneventfully.

The anxiety seemed to have decreased considerably. She talked mostly about her recent dates. She spoke freely about her apprehensions, but was well aware of her feminine emotions and desires. Her feelings about termination were discussed extensively, reactivating some of her ambivalent inclinations at the time of her father's departure. The psychotherapy had lasted four months and ended uneventfully.

Discussion

Technically, this case presented several difficulties to the therapist. I have already commented on our initial impression about her intelligence and her motivation to understand herself, but her conviction of female superiority loomed to the male therapist as a potential stumbling block. Faced during the second interview with her initial demands for a change in the appointment time and before the therapeutic alliance had a chance to develop, he was unsure how his refusal to meet this request would affect the subsequent course of psychotherapy. Silence at that point seemed to have been his best ally, and it seemed to have worked temporarily. Encouraged by this initial success the therapist proceeded to deal with the transference feelings early by referring to the patient's derogatory attitude to him. It has been stated in the chapter on technique that the transference is dealt with quite early in short-term anxiety-provoking psychotherapy. In this instance the therapist went after it relentlessly even at the risk of annoying the patient, because he sensed that the patient was exaggerating somewhat her mother's superiority over her father, and because she herself had challenged him about reading the record. The patient responded to this by becoming introspective and granting him that his logic made sense, but she returned immediately to her initial demand for a change in the hour. Now again the therapist was being challenged, and a false move on his part could mean the premature end of the treatment. He thought however that he had no alternative but to take a firm stand. "If you want to see me," he said, "it would have to be at this hour." He was obviously taking a serious gamble because the patient could have used his intransigent attitude as an easy way out, and by refusing to accept his time, she could have ended the psychotherapy. But far from it, she not only did not put up any fight but rather seemed relieved and appeared to have welcomed his action.

This was confirmed in the following interview when her attitude had changed markedly. She smiled warmly and was willing to pursue the task of exploring her feelings for the student in the library, and in subsequent interviews the subject of her femininity, until she started to resist again and was again determined to avoid talking about it. The therapist did not let her run away, however, from this anxiety-producing area. This is an important technical aspect of this kind of psychotherapy, as has already been emphasized. Anxiety is provoked here by not letting her wander away, change the subject and avoid. By stopping the patient in her tracks, the therapist was able to help her return to the subject of her relations with men, which finally led to the complete resolution of her emotional problem.

In sum, then, her attitude about men, including her father and her therapist, seemed to have been in conflict with her feminine identification. It became clear to her that succeeding intellectually, passing the exams, did not mean giving up her femininity. Her anxiety, therefore, and the resulting phobic symptoms had served the purpose of warning her that the intellectual tendencies had the upper hand. Psychotherapy helped her to become more feminine.

We have seen in the psychiatry clinic during all these years several patients who complained of examination phobias, and the majority were females. Their psychodynamic problems were very similar. Their identification with their intellectual mothers meant to them giving up their heterosexual interests — most of these patients did very well in short-term anxiety-provoking psychotherapy. One was referred for psychoanalysis.

12

ANXIETY AND HETEROSEXUAL DIFFICULTIES

First Interview

This chapter will give a continuous and detailed account of various aspects of the treatment as they come up during certain individual sessions, so as to create a more realistic picture of the doctor-patient interaction and to describe more vividly the technique which is being used, rather than to give an overall picture, as in the three cases already discussed.

A twenty-three-year-old graduate student, after she was evaluated in the psychiatry clinic, was accepted for short-term anxiety-provoking psychotherapy. She started her first psychotherapeutic interview as follows:

Patient: Just begin?

Doctor: What is it that bothers you most and what would you like to achieve in your treatment?

Patient: I think that mainly I want to improve my relationship with men, as I thought more about it; I would also like to be able to feel comfortable in situations that are not well defined.

Doctor: So you are uncomfortable. Can you describe this feeling?

Patient: I feel very uneasy, and I begin interpreting my own behavior. I am always incapable of taking an objective viewpoint, and that makes me feel uncomfortable. In other words, I am unable to rationalize situations that are ambiguous or not well defined, I get anxious. I think that when I find myself in any situation, over and above a personal relationship, I am anxious. Unless things are well structured, I feel very uncomfortable. It is sort of an inability to let things be as they are, and my constantly wanting to structure them. I think in an interpersonal relationship, when I get a negative feedback, I start misinterpreting and it makes me feel all the more uncomfortable. In my job situation I am constantly looking for answers, so this need becomes satisfied.

Doctor: Could you describe the feeling of being uncomfortable? What is it like?

Patient: It's just a very anxious feeling — it is a tight, uncanny, shaky feeling inside — and that is the only way I can describe it. It's not a fear, except perhaps maybe rejection would enter into it in some way. It's just sort of a tight feeling inside. Sometimes I just don't know exactly what I should do next, what I should say next, what topic I should choose.

The therapist gets nowhere in pursuing this line of inquiry about feelings and decides to find out something about the patient's fantasies.

Doctor: Any thoughts in your mind at that time?

Patient: I think sometimes that the thoughts which come to mind are attempts to figure out exactly what I should do — ways to structure the situation immediately. If I'm removed from the other person, like when I'm having a relationship with somebody that is ending, I'm reduced to saying, "I wish this unpleasantness would go away." Within a short period of time I'm capable of suppressing the whole thing, and after awhile it doesn't bother me any more. The relationship is no longer there. I am completely able to meet it, deal with it, and end it.

Doctor: Can you give an example?

Again the therapist gets nowhere, so he tries a different, a more concrete approach.

Patient: Well, you know when I came originally to the clinic, talking to Dr. R., when I was telling him about the last person I had gone out with on dates — a person whose background was vastly different from mine — he was not supportive of my needs. It was an impossible situation. I can remember that toward the time of termination of the relationship, instead of realizing that it was not going to work out, I took no active steps to sever the relationship, but I behaved in such a way as to make him end it. I had to know whether this person would call me again. I'd get all this situation so well defined that in a few days or a few weeks, a relationship which went on for months became no longer meaningful. It no longer made any sense. As I cut my feelings off, all the anxiety diminished. When, a month and a half later, I saw him again at a social gathering, there was just absolutely nothing left. It didn't even bother me to see him. I didn't even feel uncomfortable. It was as though he didn't and had never really existed in my mind. I would speak to him, and I could be very objective.

Doctor: Why is that a problem?

Patient: Well, the problem — no, you said to cite an example. This was an example of my personal relationships. It was well established. It was the same pattern with about six different people for maybe three years. I doubt that this control is a good thing. I'm just uncomfortable about it, and I even have fears of entering into other relationships because of it. This is what I've come to find out. Why is it happening?

Doctor: What comes to mind?

Patient: You mean, why is it happening?

Doctor: No, I said what comes to mind.

Patient: I think basically these people are very different from me. Perhaps . . . I discussed it with my mother once, and she agreed with me — I don't think I've ever dated anyone who is ready for a long-term relationship, you know, end up with marriage. When I look at my parents, I don't want the kind of marriage that they had. It reinforces my attraction for people who are completely different from them. And yet knowing all this stuff just doesn't change my attitude.

Doctor: What is the matter with your parents' marriage?

Patient: From my viewpoint? I just don't think they are happy. I know they weren't happy in the past when I lived at home. I don't think either of them feels himself as a person. My mother does maybe in some ways, but my father is not an introspective person. I see them as very good people; as individuals, I enjoy being with them — perhaps I enjoy my mother a little bit more than my father, but I'd much rather see them alone than together. I always feel like they are pulling me, to one side or the other. Yet when we're alone my mother doesn't really try so much to influence me against my father. My father is probably the one who has a more adult attitude. Together they pull against each other, and they pull my brother and me to either side. You know, either active or passive. I feel whenever I'm with them together that they're divided.

Doctor: Your brother is younger?

Patient: Yes. Five years.

Doctor: You say you are closer to your mother?

Patient: I am closer to my mother. My father doesn't question what I do. He's either delighted, or he doesn't like what I do, but he doesn't question my motives for doing anything. My mother and I can talk to each other. I go to my father for material things, but at the same time I know my parents both think that I'm wonderful. They always supported me. I haven't actually lived at home for some time.

Doctor: But how were you getting along when you were growing up?

Patient: I can't remember ever that our family was very peaceful. I used to think our family was terrible. When other people . . . I mean I used to think that what happened was disastrous . . . I know it wasn't. My father provided a good living, everything in that area was fine, but there were a lot of fights. They were bickering all the time. Probably that influenced me. I don't know how much, but it did.

Since questions about her past history seem to be productive the therapist decides to pursue this kind of questioning.

Doctor: Just for my information, let's review your background. You were born where?

Patient: Atlanta, Georgia.

Doctor: How old are you?

Patient: Twenty-three.

Doctor: Were you brought up in Atlanta also?

Patient: Yes. I lived in the same house for eighteen years.

Doctor: Going back to your early childhood, what do you remember? For instance, before your brother was born?

Patient: I was the center of attention. I don't remember any conflict. My father was very fond of me. When my brother was born, I don't think I liked him. Of course, we fought a lot. We are two different people, yet at the same time we are very close.

Doctor: Do you remember what your reaction was when you found out that you had a brother?

Patient: All I can remember is that my mother's parents took care of me. I remember one time my grandmother was teasing my father about liking my brother better. That was, I guess, when I was about seven or eight.

Doctor: Did your father say that he liked your brother best?

Patient: No, but I heard also my mother mention it to my father. I guess she said something like, "Maybe you're showing favoritism," or something like that. That's the only incident that I remember.

Doctor: You seem to say that your father's attitude changed from being attached to you to being more attached to your brother.

Patient: I viewed it this way. It . . .

Doctor: It may not really be the case?

Patient: I don't think my father is more attached to my brother. In many respects I can't explain why, but my father thinks everything I do is great, but I get nervous when I am with him. He has more criticism for my brother's behavior nowadays than he ever did for mine. I can't remember under what conditions I said it, but I can remember telling him very distinctly that I thought he preferred my brother. My father denied it. Whether I was using it to get something or other, I don't know.

Doctor: You say that your grandmother as well as your mother mentioned it.

Patient: My mother is a very mediating person. She likes things very easy. My father's very volatile and flares up easily. I feel at times very uncomfortable, so I intellectualize.

Doctor: Do you think that your father was . . .

Patient (interrupting): Likes my brother better? Maybe he does.

Doctor: No, I didn't mean that at all. I wanted to say that your father liked you possibly more than your brother, but because he even dared to show interest in someone else, this made you jealous.

This was not meant as a clarification, but rather to test the patient's reaction.

Patient: Maybe. That's quite conceivable. Perhaps after being top dog in the family, and not only in the family, but with everybody . . . I was the only grandchild, too. I had this whole contingent of worshippers.

It is obvious that the patient takes the doctor's remarks in her stride.

Doctor: Your grandparents lived close by?

Patient: Not too far — about forty miles. My mother comes from a very large family, of about eight children. A few months after I was born my cousins started coming along. But I was always the oldest and I think this added prestige . . . They lived in a farm.

Doctor: But you don't remember any specific events, such as . . .

Patient (interrupting): You mean, like actually trying to get rid of my brother?

Doctor: No, I didn't mean that. Did you have any such thoughts?

It is the therapist here who is taken aback.

Patient: I can't remember having any such thoughts. But I was sure I resented a lot the attention that was paid to my brother. He was sick, and he had to return to the hospital, and the family routine was upset. Over and above this, it was touch and go for a while whether he was going to live or not. That's the only thing I can remember about my brother when he was a baby. Only, another thing was that my brother was an extremely beautiful child. He was magnificent, and I went into this ugly period at age five or six, and when I looked at the pictures, I saw this darling baby and this ugly girl.

Doctor: Really?

Patient: Well, my mother always said the process of maturation made for change. You know this was always true. I still, in many ways, have very poor self-confidence, and it was all based in many ways on my physical beauty — sort of lack of it. You see pictures and my teeth would be out . . . there are relatively few pictures of my family that didn't show this. And always in contrast to my brother.

Doctor: You said your physical beauty and then change it to lack . . .

Patient (interrupting): I meant that I was ugly.

Doctor: Yet you said beauty. Anyway this thought of being ugly occurred to you at that time?

Patient: It occurred to me even as I was growing up. I looked at those pictures, and my brother was the star. I was cute also as a baby, but I don't think I was as cute as my brother.

Doctor: Did it occur to you that your father's attitude might have changed for any other reason?

Patient: You mean, he might have liked my brother better because he was sick or better looking? No, that never occurred to me consciously. I had this very imaginary world when I was a child.

Doctor: What kind?

Patient: I can remember mother saying that I had this imaginary planet for a while. I used to read all these fairy tales. Great fantasy world and images. I read every fairy tale that was available in our library when I was a youngster. I was a very prolific reader and devoured ten books in two weeks.

Doctor: At five you couldn't have read all that.

Patient: I could read when I was even in the first grade. I remember reading a great deal later on. We had a school library, even there, down South.

Doctor: So we can say, then, that things really changed drastically in many ways after your brother was born. Whether this was true or not as far as your father was concerned is another matter, we do not know. But the fact remains that you had the impression that this was the case.

You also say you changed in appearance. A few years later you accused your father of being not interested in you. You became a prolific reader, with a fantasy world of your own. How did things develop after that?

Patient: I was a discipline problem in grade school. You mean, like after I went to school? Well, my family was very religious. My brother and I were baptized as Episcopalians, and he always practiced this religion. I stopped practicing mine. I remember I did something in the classroom, and I wasn't allowed to go to church with the group and finally I had to go separately — all by myself. This was very disturbing. I just hated the church. When I had to go by myself, I was just terrified. Somehow, I guess I figured that if I went with the rest of the children it was going to be easier, but . . . well, I started to make trouble at school. I was always in with these people who were disturbing things in the classroom. Even in the first grade one of the boys stole something, I don't remember what, and of course the whole class was censured by the teacher immediately. I took his side, and she was mad. Then there were a couple of incidents when I stole things myself. I was always caught, but nothing drastic happened. I was always at the nucleus of the activities. I was always involved in making trouble. I was totally uninterested in school in what was going on in the classroom. Except maybe geography, but nothing to do with arithmetic. I always hated it. English was fine. I liked that. But when it got so that whenever anything went wrong, whether I was involved or not, I was always picked up. I remember my mother had to go down and talk with the principal, but it was different outside the school situation. I was never in trouble with the police. It always had to do with the school, when these things would happen. Always having to sit in the wardrobe.

Doctor: When did all this happen?

Patient: All the way through, right up to the eighth grade. I got thrown out of the choir in eighth grade, just in time for the dedication of the new school. I even wrote the constitution for the class, and I made a lot of noise. Then it all stopped when I was in high school. I was never on detention. I never was in trouble. I think a lot of it was that my reputation sort of followed me from grade school and everybody expected that I might cause a lot of trouble, but I didn't.

Doctor: Could it be that something happened?

Patient: Something that I didn't like in school?

Doctor: In you.

Patient: In me? . . . Between the time I left eighth grade and went into high school? Nothing happened other than that I left the school and changed to another school. I don't remember anything significant.

Doctor: Something physical, for instance?

Patient: Like menstruating? I started my menstrual cycle in the seventh grade. I was very well prepared for it. My mother was the one who prepared me for it. I gained other kinds of knowledge from outside, but the initial contact came from her. She is a very frank person. These kinds of things didn't upset her.

Doctor: I was more interested whether they upset you.

Patient: Oh no, not at all.

Doctor: It seems quite clear that instead of your being upset, you settled down. Is this the time you have talked about some kind of reaction? You were rebellious, you were doing things to antagonize the teachers, and then suddenly you change, you settle down, and you describe that all was going along very well.

Patient: Well, don't get the wrong impression. I didn't follow rules or anything. My whole theory developed as follows: You don't get up there and you don't protest against things violently, because it doesn't work that way. You work hard and you get certain advantages and then you have them taken away. "No, I said to myself, that is not the way." I became much more confident. I can remember certain kids actively agitating and campaigning. "Let's all change the rules," they said, and I can remember thinking, "This is ridiculous, because you can always get around the rules." So, in other words, maybe my values became more subversive — I did not take action. I learned to get around the rules.

Doctor: What happened to this rebellion at the present time? Did it vanish?

Patient: I'm just not an active rebel. Maybe I will voice my opinion very strongly about people that I think are not in a position to threaten me. If they're in any position to threaten me, they just don't find out about it, because I do not express how I feel about them. I would never go to the administration or the chairman of my department and say, "I don't like the way you people teach; we're going to change all this." I am not an activist, but I certainly can talk around various people in authority. To people who are under me, or to my contemporaries, I can express how I feel. I can say, "I don't like this, that, or the other thing." But as far as the authorities are concerned, I have a whole different way of operating, which has become very rational — a calm type of a "thing." Every time I have something to say I think of three thousand five hundred reasons. I have it all figured out. I can get around them.

Doctor: You mean, you use your intellect to deal with subversion?

Patient: I guess so.

Doctor: You know, you did the same thing here. As you discussed your problem with men, you presented it in a very clinical, intellectual, and roundabout way.

Patient: Of course; but, as I said, I feel bad about doing this. I can look at it objectively. I can deal with it. Actually, it's very disturbing. It's not as comfortable as I make it sound. You could not rationalize all the time. It just does not change the basic feeling. And this is the most frustrating thing. You are going to have to live with it gracefully, or some kind of change is going to have to take place. At school, I can use my subversive techniques. I wouldn't even feel sad if the chairman of my department said that he was going to expel me or something. I would get around that sort of thing. Anyway I know that I am very competent in what I'm doing. It's just when it gets into this other area. With my boy friends there's no relationship at all. I am a competent machine. Many people say that I don't give myself credit for what I do, yet I don't have any self-confidence.

Doctor: Going back to the subversion or the rebellion — what were you rebelling against?

Patient: Problems at home. My father and mother started to fight. It seems that their relationship disintegrated. My mother should have gotten a divorce. I remember I used to think I did not want to go with my mother if she divorced my father. I used to think it was preferable for my mother to pack and go. She was the disciplinarian. I can manipulate my father. He is easier to get along with. I can get all the money from him. I can reason with him. Yet, in other ways, my mother is more adaptable than my father. She is like me.

Doctor: Or the other way around.

Patient: . . . Yes, I see what you mean. Well, anyway, I could not see that there was any love between them.

The interview continued with more history-taking, which covered her years at college.

A description of the patient's physical appearance may be in order at this point. She was a tall, dark-haired woman, with blue eyes. She gave an over-all impression of being masculine. She wore pants and combed her long hair close to her head. She wore a suede jacket. The predominating coloring was grey-blue. Her shoes were flat. There was a warm smile which appeared occasionally and would light up her face, but most of the time she frowned, looked quizzical, and showed only a pained and anxious expression.

Before the end of the interview it seemed that a decision had to be made as to the area of emotional conflict to concentrate upon and to try to understand during the psychotherapy. In the therapist's opinion the patient's difficulty with men and her anxiety and tension associated with it, which she handled by intellectualizing, rationalizing, and controlling, seemed to be similar to the way she handled her father. After the birth of her brother, and after her so-called demotion to a position of being second-best, which she attributed to being feminine and ugly, a period of rebellion ensued, which was followed after puberty by quiet subversion in the form of manipulating men and evading her feelings for them. Dissatisfied and curious, she came to the clinic for help. Her difficulty with men, which could be traced to her relation with her father, was the emotional problem to be investigated and solved during the therapy. This formulation was presented to the patient, who readily agreed.

Second Interview

Patient: Shall I start where we left off? (Without waiting for an answer): You were asking me questions about my family life and things at home. I remember you were asking me about how I felt about my parents' quarreling when I was a child and whom I wanted to stay with if they divorced. (Pause.) Then we decided to look into all the problems I had with young men which were similar to the problems I had with my father. I gave it some thought and I agree it is important. Where shall I start?

Doctor: You may talk about anything you wish, as long as it has something to do with the problem we have outlined.

Patient: I do? (Laughing.)

Doctor: This is *your* hour.

Patient: Well, the thing that I thought about most was how I feel, rather than how I talk or think. Several times you asked me how I felt about things, and I came out with the big intellectual "thing" as an answer. I do just this sort of thing to hide the way I feel. In other words, I try to smooth things out. Also, I sort of control people by intellectualizing. I am using this "mind thing" . . .

Doctor: Why is it that you use this "mind thing," as you put it?

Although the therapist has an opportunity to pick the transference issue, he decides to follow the patient's lead.

Patient: Because I think that's the best way to manipulate people and to get what I want from them. I tried not to do it this weekend, but it didn't work out. I went down to New York for a meeting, and this whole issue came up about changing hotels. This time I made a huge issue out of it all. It was important that we were all in the same hotel, plus the fact that I wanted a friend of mine to stay with me. I raised so much fuss — I talked and argued — but, of course, because there was a convention it had absolutely no effect whatsoever. It didn't change the way things happened. I don't think I felt any better after shouting about it, and after making a big scene and being more aggressive. I think I would have done better if I tried to discuss things reasonably.

Doctor: I am not sure that I know exactly what happened.

Patient: We got down to the New York hotel, and we had three rooms reserved, one month in advance. Usually hotels overbook their reservations. It became clear that they were not about to honor our reservations. Of course, we weren't the only ones. There was a gigantic line of people. Usually when I get mad I start discussing things rationally, and I succeed. I usually make my point clear. When I succeed I just forget about it. This time I demanded to see the assistant manager, and I was quite firm. I said that we weren't going to stay at another hotel unless they paid our transportation back and forth. I told him that their public relations were very poor. You know — I said that with a lot of force — with much more emotional content than I am describing to you now, but it didn't change the situation a bit, and I didn't feel any better for doing it. He did get mad, however.

Doctor: Why did you feel that you had to change the way you do things?

Patient: I thought it would get me what I wanted, if I put more feeling into it instead of being just cold, intellectualizing . . . (pause). Perhaps when people are emotional, like the manager, I am more inclined to come across. If they present some rational plan — if they are bland — it removes the vehemence of my response . . . (pause).

Doctor: Did you think that I want you to be more emotional?

Patient: Oh, no. No, I felt that I wanted to try it . . . (pause).

Doctor: You emphasized that I asked you about how you felt. From what follows the transference issue is a bit premature.

Patient (paying no attention): We also talked about — I mean I talked about being able to cope with ambiguous relationships. I have become more and more aware — I don't know if this is just because I have been talking about it lately — but the whole problem seems to be very important. Somehow being calm and reasonable in the face of an emotional storm and not getting carried away, except for last weekend, is my customary way of dealing with people. I am sure that this calm exterior of mine is *abnormal.*

Doctor: Your emphasis is impressive . . . All this intellectualizing of yours is a way of dealing with your feelings. It represents a solution to a problem. The question is, whether it is a good solution for you or not.

Patient (paying no attention): Is it just all right if I ramble on about anything? Do you want me to talk about this problem? Can I just put things together?

Doctor: This is your therapy, and you can do whatever you want to do with it, but I am intrigued by your question. Is it a way to avoid my question?

Patient: Oh, no. It is just that this weekend I came across this realization. All of a sudden I discovered I wanted all this power. It was sort of an overwhelming discovery because it was so sudden — I guess I thought that women are not supposed to be power-hungry and they are not supposed to have strengths or to have asocial desires. This violent way of acting is not acceptable in our culture, and this was impressed upon me when I grew up. Anyway, I got this tremendous urge to promote my own status. Actually, I just felt magnificent — this meeting I attended in New York was a very important one for my career. I was very fortunate in having met some very fine people. I really got a taste of it. I really liked it. At times I have this sort of conflict, on the one hand I have the self-confidence to do what I want, but most often what stops me usually is this poor image of myself.

Doctor: Since you say you have a poor image of yourself, why do you have it?

Patient: I don't know why. Sometimes I have no self-confidence at all. It's getting a little better, or maybe it's coming out a little more in subtle ways. I don't know, but I do devaluate myself a lot. Inside me there are things which I am afraid to face . . .

Doctor: Again, the question is, why do you? I don't expect an answer to this question. What I mean is, what comes to mind? Why do you have to overcompensate for it, which is a solution, as I said before. Is it a good one?

Patient: I don't know why I feel that way. I just do.

Doctor: Is this, then, another aspect which we may consider worth trying to understand in your psychotherapy? As I see it, in the hotel episode you had no alternative.

Here the therapist introduces a secondary emotional problem to be solved, namely the patient's poor image of herself, which is clearly linked with the original problem of her relations with men.

Patient: In the hotel I put on a temper tantrum, but I realized clearly that I had no alternative. The writing was on the wall. We had to move. I had to accept it without volition.

Doctor: Was it then the best place to express your feelings, when the failure was inevitable?

Patient: Well, it was safer for me to act it out there than some other place.

Doctor: Now, let us look at this example, for instance. There was nothing you could do at the hotel. It was not the best place to have your temper tantrum, and maybe the intellectualized approach would have been better under the circumstances. In another situation, however, when you can change things, when it is in your hands to be more forthright, it may be different. These are ways you use to handle the problem of inadequacy. What is quite clear is that at times you do have feelings of inadequacy; yet, at the same time, as you have told me, you are a very competent and power-hungry person. These two attitudes are in conflict with each other. The question we still have is: why do you have this poor image of yourself and why are you power-hungry? Where do these attitudes come from?

Patient: I don't know, because I haven't thought about where it comes from. It just exists.

Doctor: This is just as good a time as any to start thinking. What comes to your mind?

The therapist decides that it is about time to start asking anxiety-provoking questions.

Patient (pause): In terms of what I feel, about this poor self-confidence? I view myself as being different from what I want to be.

Doctor: That's all intellectual, and you know it.

Patient (irritably): All I can say is that I set these things up, that I think they are very important, and, as you know, I want these things; but at the same time I feel I'll never attain them. I like to intellectualize. I don't know where to start about finding out why I feel this way.

Doctor: What comes to mind about it?

Patient: For heaven's sake . . . (blushing). I — just sort of feel blah . . . I don't know how to describe these feelings. I don't like it. I just don't like these feelings. They're distasteful. I don't like your questions.

Doctor: Distasteful. You don't like them. Blah. Under what circumstances do you have such feelings?

Patient: It depends on the circumstances. I admire people who are very bright. When I came to this part of the country, I realized intellectuality was very important, but when I went to college it was the other way around. The emphasis was not on using your brain in any way at all. A southern belle — you know, all that nonsense. It's not just *one* thing that makes me feel inadequate. Can't you see? When I was in college it was social situations. Now I feel it's intellectual situations. I don't feel like I should take over a conversation when a person is bright. Sometimes I feel as if I don't have anything to say that's going to be particularly brilliant. This upsets me. When I came here, I met a completely different type of people who were totally different from what I encountered in Atlanta. Over there anyone who did any reading was out of it. The group of people I went around with were very socially inclined. In other words, I sort of incorporated their values into mine. I still think those things are important, but other things opened up when I came up North. It's not that I don't think it's important to be socially popular. I place a great deal of importance on dates and things like that, but the intellectual atmosphere up here is different . . . I had never been exposed to these things (long pause). Maybe, in a sense, my standards are unrealistic for my ability. I've tried to look realistically at what I'm capable of, but I don't have any reference point except down below my standards. I don't see myself as approaching them. I have this very strong feeling: the best or nothing at all. Throw it away.

Doctor: What do you mean, down below?

Patient: What I've set is sort of perfectionism, as being desirable. I see myself as being way below this high standard. I look down there, and I see nothing.

Doctor: Can you tell me a little bit more about this feeling "down below"?

Patient: It doesn't have to do with any one particular thing. It is not important. It has to do with what I set out as desirable as far as . . .

The therapist is aware that she is trying to avoid his question.

Doctor: You are already in the process of devaluing your statement. You made a statement which is of interest. Then I ask you about it, and you say it isn't important. Now let's get back to it.

Patient: About what these standards are?

Doctor: Of being below . . . these standards, if you like . . .

Patient: Well, I don't feel like I am approaching them. I feel that all these things are magnificent. I want to attain these things; but I feel I lack something, and then I don't want them any more for fear of failure. I feel myself not capable. I've always coped with the situation. I have to be realistic. I do find that I understand somebody who comes up to me and says, "I want to do this and that, but I'll just never achieve it." I know exactly what they are talking about.

Doctor: You seem to be saying that you lack something. What does that feeling remind you of?

Patient: What do you mean? The feeling that I lack something reminds me of something? It doesn't remind me of anything; it's a negative state. I'm not happy that way, and I haven't accepted my limitations. But I . . .

Doctor: Yes, I can see this. I know you don't like it. But what does it bring to mind from the past? Where does this come from?

Patient (pause): I've always — I can remember feeling this way in high school. Do you mean how far back have I felt this way — being incompetent? For as long as I can remember. Right when I was back in grade school. I can remember being on the outside group. Like, in high school it wasn't like being in the outside group, but in not being with the leaders of the school. I just never would accept the responsibility to go out and do anything by myself. I expected that I would always be disappointed. These wishes were always substituted by something else, which was always not quite as desirable . . . I was lonely.

Doctor: So, since this is something that has been going on for a long period of time, we must try to find its origin way back.

Patient: Oh, I think so, but why would I feel this way when I was younger?

Doctor: That's a good question.

Patient: All the things I can think of seem like intellectual illusions. Well, as we were talking before — maybe because I was the center of attention and after my brother came I felt I was outside the family circle. Up to the time my brother arrived in the family I was the center of attention, but I can't remember feeling that way as strongly as I feel now.

Doctor: What aspect of the problem makes you feel strongly now?

Patient: About being on the outside of the family? No, no. I don't think in terms of it now. Actually, I am in a more favorable position than my brother at the present time. He isn't threatening me at all now, whereas then he may have been a rival. Now I don't feel threatened by him at all. It's possibly transferred to other things.

Doctor: There's a paradox in what you are saying. You say that at the time you were not particularly aware of it, yet now, on thinking about it, you feel strongly.

Patient: No, no. I told you that anything I thought sounds psychological or reasonable. I can't remember how I felt then, except that I remember seeing the nurse with my brother, and that we always fought a lot. I don't think that was particularly abnormal, but maybe it was.

Doctor: You think it felt distasteful, "blah"?

The doctor is too eager here to tie things together and on the surface seems to fail.

Patient: No, I don't remember feeling that way at all. I

don't remember how I really felt. Just flashes of memory come back. Visual things. There doesn't seem to be any feeling connected with it (pause). I think the first strong feelings I had about being incompetent were when it came to dating. Because as a child . . . well, no, no, it came when I saw these pictures; no, it must have come with dating and the idea that I was very tall — in the seventh and eighth grade I was the same height as I am now — I had these gigantic feet, and I hated wearing orthopedic shoes. The whole thing was disgusting. I blamed all these various things for my unpopularity, and I can remember my mother saying, "It will all end" — you know, in other words, "Just wait this out," but I just didn't see things this way at all. (Her face had a pained expression.)

The patient is trying hard to disentangle her memories and her feelings.

Doctor: So this feeling has something to do with physical appearance?

Patient: Yeah, maybe it does have something to do . . . yeah, sure. But it has to do with intellectual competency, too. (She grimaced and looked sad.)

Doctor: Let's go back for a minute. What about this physical appearance?

Patient: That wasn't important.

Doctor: There you are trying to deny what you just said. But it is important now. I can see it. Furthermore your behavior betrays it. As you were talking about it your facial expression changed. You looked sad. Now, about your reaction to being very tall. You showed a lot of feeling. Can you tell me something about it?

Patient: I can remember that. Very vividly!

Doctor: So the feeling is present right now as well as at that time. Yet you tried to run away from it.

Patient: No, yeah, right.

Doctor: Yes or no?

Patient: Yes, yes.

Doctor: Let's hear about it then.

Patient: About the visual picture — about how I looked? About these feelings that I had when I was younger? . . .

(expecting an answer) . . . Well . . . I can always remember having to be last in line because I was so tall and also because my name came last. I used to joke about it, but I didn't like it. I was very sensitive because I always had to stand at the end of the line all the time. There was another girl who was sort of with me, but still I was the tallest until I graduated. Finally other kids caught up with me. But this was very . . . in the fifth and sixth and seventh grades, from when I was ten on up, I was standing at the end of the line. I considered myself this "gigantic thing." In pictures, I can remember when I was in the sixth grade we had this group picture, and I just didn't like the idea of being so tall, so I just sort of bent down to be the same height as everybody else. In church processions I was always at the end of the line. I can remember I didn't like the way I looked, but I think this had more to do with looking at those pictures that were taken of me when I was in kindergarten. I had no teeth, and physically I was an awful looking sight. In contrast my brother was beautiful, magnificent. I mean physically. He was just a beautiful baby, while at that time I was sort of incongruous, ridiculous. Then I went through this period of gaining weight. I swam an awful lot. Physically, I was always well coordinated. My brother was always very uncoordinated. And this was always very important to me. I remember gaining a lot of weight when I was sixteen because I stopped doing all these things. I stopped dancing, and I just sort of gave all these activities up; so, added to this gigantic height, I gained weight. My mother didn't seem to be too concerned about this at all. I was far more concerned about it. She never, as far as I can remember, ever said anything about losing weight, or changing things around, or made any comments at all. I for one, felt this very strongly. Not that any of my friends said anything, but I was very conscious of being apart from others at school.

Doctor: Isn't it peculiar that no one seemed to have paid attention to this incongruous sight? What was your father's attitude?

Patient: He never said a word, I don't remember him getting involved in this at all.

Doctor: Not at all?

Patient: Well, I don't remember. I never talked to my father about this thing. After I was in the fifth grade, I didn't talk to my father about anything at all. I never said a word, for example, about being fat or anything else. Unless my mother told him. I can remember telling my mother these things.

Doctor: But isn't there something peculiar in all this? You have strong feelings. You talk to your mother, and you find your mother not concerned. Why don't you talk to your father?

Patient: Well, I don't see why . . . I don't remember talking to him at all. I don't remember discussing anything like that with him. If it was strange, I never remember carrying it past that. I guess going to my mother was far enough. Unless of course that at the time I wasn't interested in talking to my father. I mean he was — this to me was a female thing — I just couldn't see where he would be interested in it.

Doctor: That's an interesting way of looking at it. Doesn't your appearance have something to do with men?

Patient: Right, but somehow Daddy was never involved in that.

Doctor: I don't think you involved him.

Patient: I didn't, no. I didn't involve him. That was about the time . . . my mother was the one who gave me my sexual education . . . and I talked to her about these things.

Doctor: Yes. And you told me that your mother didn't help you out in this situation.

Patient: Well, what was she going to do? It wasn't that she wasn't concerned. She just never said anything. She was not nagging, "Go on a diet," and stuff like this. I would come to her with these things, and she would be very, very calm and we would discuss it in terms of the problem. It wasn't just that I was turned off.

Doctor: Maybe your mother wanted you to get fat.

Patient: Well, I — maybe she did. My mother's very good looking. I don't see why my attractiveness either one way or the other would pose any problems for her.

Doctor: No?

Patient: At times I've thought about it. Not that I . . . that all mothers went through a stage when they set themselves up in competition with their daughters — I'm sure I went through this.

Doctor: Of course it could be the other way around.

Patient: I don't remember feeling this way, outside of the fact that there came a time when I was no longer — did not appear without clothes on, in front of my father. I was very conscious about that.

Doctor: Hmm. When was that?

Patient: Probably about that time when I was . . . about five or so. From then on and particularly in the sixth grade and on up I didn't talk to him. That's when I seemed to favor talking to my mother. Now the idea of my setting myself up, of being a threat to my mother — this is something I reasoned out myself. This is a very normal thing. I couldn't consider myself a threat to my mother — I mean, considering the way I looked! I find it very hard to see. I mean, now I could be a greater threat to my mother than I was when I was in the fifth and sixth grade . . .

Doctor: Are you now?

Patient: I don't want to place myself in this position — in *her* position. I am more independent than my mother — more intellectual.

Doctor: Did you become intellectual because you could not compete with your mother physically? You say she was beautiful and you were ugly.

Patient: I do not know. My mother had a very active social life before she got married . . . She talked about it, and it was very boring to me. Lots and lots of men, lots of dates, and stuff like that, going out a lot to parties. She was very happy at that time in contrast to being unhappy in her marriage. They fouled things up when they got married. She was extremely attractive and dressed very well. She also had a terrific imagination . . . she was very happy.

Doctor: Was she sexual?

Patient: No, no. Not really — she was very attractive to men, but I never thought of sexual intercourse. I *never, never* thought of my mother in that role. I never thought of my parents having sexual intercourse. I suppose I suppressed it religiously.

Doctor: You did, did you!

Patient: Oh, yes. But, mind you, it was about *them* not about . . . I mean I had sexual thoughts all right.

Doctor: Now isn't there something odd in all this?

Patient: What do you mean? Oh, no, no. I am sure my mother was very innocent. She didn't have any sexual thoughts, I am sure of that.

Doctor: You are sure, are you? I think you are sure you had sexual thoughts. You were sure you thought your mother did not have sexual thoughts, but you do not *know* whether she did or not. Miss W., I do not think you want to know.

It may appear that the therapist is inconsistent during this hour. He does not seem to pursue any definite line of inquiry. Although the transference comes up repeatedly in terms of questions from the patient as to procedure, he decides to ignore them. This he does on purpose, because the patient uses formidable intellectualized defenses. One may describe his technique as trying to take the patient by surprise and to bypass her attempts to control the therapeutic situation. Having failed repeatedly he is rewarded with valuable information about the patient's body image and, more importantly, he is able to see that she has strong feelings in this area which are available to be examined during the interview. Finally all this leads to the emergence of a vivid picture of the patient's interaction with her parents.

This purposeful hit-and-miss type of interviewing has proved to be rewarding during this session. Let us see how the patient reacts to it.

Third Interview

Patient: Just start? (laugh) (pause) . . .

Doctor: Why do you hesitate? You want some guidance?

Patient: Yeah, it's just that I'm going to start (pause) . . . You just want me to keep talking about last week?

Doctor: I don't want you to do anything.

Patient: Oh! Okay. (Laughs.)

Doctor: Carry on.

Patient: Oh, well, last week we were talking about my mother, about (pause) how ugly I felt and everything. Then I talked about when I was eleven or twelve and about why I didn't discuss the same things with my father and my mother (pause) who was not concerned about my change, and maybe that she saw me in competition with her. Is this what you want to hear?

Doctor: Now what we want to understand is the way you feel. Why do you want to please me?

Patient: No, no, well, you know, it's not a question that I want to tell you something that I think you ought to hear. I don't exactly know (pause) if I just should explain all this stuff out. I mean, we seemed to be talking about something completely different from the basic problem I brought. Now I feel it's important but —

Doctor: Which one now?

Patient: Well, the original problem we decided to solve. The problem about my relations with other people — with men.

Doctor: You don't think the subject we talked about last week has anything to do with your interpersonal relationships?

Patient: Oh! I do think the way I feel about the way I look is very important.

Doctor: It is also important how you handled your appearance in terms of your parents . . . and

Patient: Oh, you mean my parents' attitude toward the way I felt about the way I looked?

Doctor: How *you* felt about it, and how it affected your relations with your parents. We saw that there were certain differences as far as your father and your mother were concerned. Weren't there? Doesn't that have something to do with interpersonal relations?

Patient: No, that's right; but I don't see that it makes any difference, because my father wasn't ever involved. In other words, maybe I had a special attitude about the way I felt he was reacting, but in reality I don't remember him saying

237

anything. I knew my father had certain standards that were set, but they had nothing to do with the way I looked or the way I dressed (laughing). Maybe I'm just not aware of anything about how my father might have felt; I know how I felt about my father. Of course, I forgot about my mother. I don't know what I talked about.

Doctor: You seem to be forgetting today all over the place. Is it a reaction to last week's hour?

Patient: You know, there was something about my mother that we talked — that I talked about, but . . . Oh, yes, it was her being attractive . . . and all that stuff about sex. Well, I felt very upset being in the middle when my parents were arguing, but I also seemed to love it.

From then on the major part of the interview was spent on the patient's description of her parents' quarrels, and of how she became aware of her enjoyment in being the center of attention. She also described how she had used one of her boy friends, whom her parents disliked, in such a way as to precipitate a quarrel between her parents and then she sat back and watched them all perform. She said that she felt happy and somewhat guilty about having been able to use her boy frient Mort as "a pawn." She finally talked about feeling lonely.

It seems clear that the patient during this hour is trying to run away from what she talked about and experienced during the second interview. This is understandable, and although the therapist points to her covering up maneuvers, he is not too insistent. The patient worked very hard. She needs some rest. A pause seems necessary.

Fourth Interview

The patient came ten minutes late for this interview and started by saying:

Patient: I have nothing to say. I felt that I should prepare myself. I feel ill at ease talking about all this . . .

Doctor: About what apsect of all this?

Patient: I don't feel comfortable. Maybe I intellectualize to avoid talking about what counts . . . I felt lonely this week. It is an unpleasant feeling when I am lonely. I feel a need to do something — to act in some way to get out of it.

Doctor: Will action solve the way you feel?

Patient: No.

Doctor: What makes you feel this way?

Patient (impatiently): I don't know. I feel and I felt uncomfortable this whole week. I didn't feel like being with people. I've been very negative all this week. I don't like to be directed by anyone in any way. Yet I feel so alone.

Doctor: Do you think that these feelings have to do with your psychotherapy?

Since the transference has more or less been avoided up to now, the therapist thought that it was time to bring it into the open before it developed into a resistance. He may not have pursued vigorously enough, however, the need of the patient to act in some way to avoid her loneliness, and he may regret it.

Patient: No.

Doctor: With me?

Patient: No. It's that I don't feel like myself today.

Doctor: Is this why you were ten minutes late?

Patient: Oh, no, no . . .

She then spent considerable time giving the reasons why she was late, but she was able to see that there was something she was avoiding.

Patient: I don't know why I feel this way and why I felt this way the whole week.

Doctor: Does it have something to do with the last interview?

Patient: Maybe . . . I hate it when I feel that I must perform.

Doctor: So you want me to perform today, to do the work, and ask you questions.

Patient: In a way you are right, yet I know it is funny. It is even ridiculous. It is like a play. I watch people perform. I guess I watch you perform, too. It is like a child playing a game — what I told you about . . .

Doctor: Hmm. It is important not to avoid your feelings about what happens here between you and me.

Patient (as if she had not heard him): I remember now. It

was so ridiculous watching all three of them perform. It was an absurd situation. They were ludicrous. I sat there unemotionally watching them. Like watching a play, I didn't get involved. In a way, it is wrong to manipulate people and to enjoy it. My father, my mother, and Mort. What a sight!

She then talked in detail about a quarrel with her mother over some clothes she bought and which her mother took back to the store because they were very expensive. She described how she was able to draw her father into the argument, how she manipulated him to take her side and give her the money, and, finally, how she went to the store, bought the same clothes back and wore them "triumphantly" in front of her mother. Then she again talked about feeling anxious and lonely.

Doctor: So loneliness follows your so-called victory, your triumph over your mother.

Patient: It is a fear of being by myself. It usually is associated with having managed people. It is the price I pay for controlling them; but it is a high price, because anxiety and loneliness are such terrible feelings.

Doctor: Although this is true and it is important for us to see the sequence, there is another aspect to these feelings which it seems to me that you missed. You know, after all, we do spend most of the time in our lives by ourselves.

Patient: Even if it is so, I haven't realized it. Maybe it is true, but it is so devastating, so bleak a perspective.

Doctor: Then it seems to me that you have not become acquainted with yourself as yet. In these efforts of yours to control people, to watch them act unemotionally and all that, you fail to discover another world — the world which exists within oneself. This world is full of fascination and excitement if one starts paying attention to it. It is full of grandiose plans, complicated solutions, magnificent scenes, terrible catastrophies, clever schemes, insoluble conflicts, and, above all, full of original thoughts and ideas which open up wide horizons of unending possibilities. There is no better spectacle than to look with our eyes open, inside our own minds. What a pity that you have missed such a grand entertainment.

Patient: You like yourself?

Doctor: . . . Yes, I do.

Patient: I guess I could like myself, too.

Doctor: Why not?

Patient: You think I could?

Doctor: I have no doubt that you can, but we must also understand not only what gets you lonely in the first place but also why you have to manage people.

Patient: Oh, I know that. It usually follows my having controlled or managed people successfully.

Doctor: People in general, and your mother in particular.

Patient: . . . Yes . . . Yes . . . it does have something to do with my mother. It is a feeling of having somehow been able to defeat her.

Doctor: You are right.

It is possible that the interview which started in a negative tone ends in a positive note, because of the transference confrontation.

Fifth Interview

Patient: I can remember all about our discussion about loneliness but I forget the rest . . . What did we talk about? I feel embarrassed . . . Oh, yes, something to do with my parents.

Doctor: Parents?

Patient: It must be very important to me if I am forgetting it . . . Nothing seems to come to my mind . . .

Doctor: How do you feel about . . .

Patient: Forgetting, yes, I know . . . I don't even think when I am in such a situation.

Doctor: How do you . . .

Patient: Feel, yes, I know . . . You asked me that . . . Well, frustrated. That's what it is; but of course when I don't think about it, it does not bother me.

Doctor: Frustrated about what?

Patient: That I can't remember the end of the last hour.

Doctor: What does it feel like not to be able to remember?

Patient: I can't remember . . . (giggling).

Doctor: It seems like a joke?

Patient: Well, no . . . but we are going around in circles.

Doctor: Yes, indeed. Are you watching the show from your detached position?

Patient (seriously): No, I don't like to do that . . . (then, looking sad:) I feel like nothing is going to help. Nothing is there. Just blah. Nothing inside. When I think about forgetting there is nothing there.

Doctor: Tell me about this "nothing there" feeling.

Patient: Empty. Nothing is inside. That's the definition of the word empty.

Doctor: Thank you, dictionary!

Patient (laughing): . . . Well, you know . . . I know (giggling) . . .

Doctor: Still amused?

Patient: Not really . . . Embarrassment . . .

Doctor: Still nothing?

Patient: I feel like an idiot because I look and there is nothing there . . . It's panic-like . . . In other situations like this one I start to talk, to say anything. I talk to cover up, to fill the gap, to pretend that I have not forgotten.

Doctor: Do you cover up now?

Patient: Oh, no, no, no. I meant in other situations. I was giving this as an example. I do cover up when I am talking, but not now . . . Now I do feel empty. Maybe this has something to do with it. Maybe I get embroiled in too many different things and then I forget.

Doctor: What you just said has nothing to do with it, and you know it.

Patient: I know it, but what can I do? . . . (silent for a long time and then, casually:) I have learned this attitude of covering up from my parents, and I blame them for it. It is their attitude not mine.

Doctor: It is not true. This is your attitude, even if you learned it from them. What do you think?

The therapist thinks it is time to start using more often anxiety-provoking confrontations.

Patient: Oh, you! (irritably): . . . It is not mine; and, further-more, I feel resentful about it, and I have this same attitude with men when I go out on dates.

Doctor: So you resent this cover-up attitude of yours which you claim that you learned from your parents and use with men on your dates.

Patient: Yes. Men are weak in my opinion. I can manipulate them. I cover up. I can do anything I want to them. Only with strong men, I do not respond this way.

Doctor: Is your father a strong or a weak man?

Patient (smiling): I wanted my way.

Doctor: Why do you smile?

Patient: I don't know. There must be something I can't remember, but consciously when I wanted something I could manipulate my father and I would get what I wanted my own way. You have a funny expression —

Doctor: I was simply asking why you smiled.

Patient: I don't know . . . There is something inside me that tries to work all these things out, all the things we are talking about. Yet the whole thing is foggy . . . You see, I feel that I didn't need their love, or something like that . . . I felt terribly rejected when I thought that my parents didn't love me, but I don't know why I was smiling.

Doctor: Unless you wanted to be rejected by only one of them.

Patient: I just wanted my father on my side. You see, my mother interfered with that . . . but you see there was no feeling about this — none at all. For example, I would think of them dying, and it didn't matter at all. I made no huge fuss about it. It wouldn't bother me for some reason or other.

Doctor: What about this thought of your parents dying?

Patient: Just that they would die, period . . . (looking abstracted and far away).

Doctor: What are you thinking about right this minute?

Patient: . . . Dying . . . I don't feel anything. I can achieve distance and dissociate myself.

Doctor: Dissociation is one of the ways to avoid feelings, indeed. There is another element in all this. You do not separate your parents. You tend to lump them together. What are your feelings about your father's or your mother's death?

Patient: I don't have any feelings, even for my brother's. It is like that whole issue of sexual relations. I never gave it a thought as far as my parents are concerned. You doubt what I say?

Doctor: No.

Patient: Oh.

Doctor: No, far from it. I am convinced.

Patient: Isn't it surprising? I never ever thought of my parents having sexual relations, because I never saw any demonstration of affection between them. What I heard was fighting. There was no semblance of any love.

Doctor: You did not see any, possibly because you did not want to see anything which you could interpret as evidence of love between your parents.

Patient: I thought more about their fighting.

Doctor: Is the thought that they loved each other threatening to you?

The therapist continues using anxiety-provoking questions which seem to lead straight into the area of the patient's conflict with her parents.

Patient: I don't know, (irritably) but I did want my father to be on my side. That I did know. When they fought I thought that my father fought with my mother because he wanted to be with me and not with her. I don't know why, since I had nothing to offer.

Doctor: Maybe you did?

The therapist does not let the patient retreat into her passive position. His question produces immediate results.

Patient: Who, me? . . . (broad smile). With fellows, maybe, this is true sometimes only.

Doctor: Can you tell me about it?

Patient (giggling): Could I! Well, when I say something clever or wear a new dress, or look at them when I feel excited . . . I use them as a means to get what I want. It's an awful thing to do — to use other people — but I do it, and I did it with my parents. Even I used my grandfather to build me up. I had nothing to give them.

Doctor: Nothing, like being empty?

Patient: What? Oh, yes. Just like before . . . But I do feel, I really do — I just need others to give me a boost — to build me up.

Doctor: You say that you had nothing to give them. You emphasize always the negative, yet we know that you have a lot to offer. Do you want to give them something?

Patient: Oh, yes. Of course . . . I have a lot to offer, for example, to people at the school. I don't get this empty feeling at school. I feel full, with a lot to give. It's on dates with the fellows that I feel empty.

Doctor: Can you give me an example?

Patient: You mean about my dating with fellows? Well, I feel sort of defective or something like that. It is at that point that I switch and then I start using the other person.

Doctor: What is it like to feel defective?

Patient: I am not sure what you mean. When I am successful?

Doctor: Just give me a simple example — not when you are successful, but when you feel defective.

Patient: Well, I don't understand.

Doctor: Come on, now Miss W. You are running away, you are avoiding. I just want you to give me an example so that we can understand what goes on.

Again the therapist presses the patient so as to avoid her running away from the subject.

Patient: . . . Well, this fellow I went out with — I destroyed the relationship on purpose. I fell in love with him, so as soon as I realized it, I thought maybe I had nothing to offer him, and the next thing I do is to forget we had a date. So I feel awful about it, I call and I apologize to him. Later on however I went on asking him what to do so he would tell me and I would not follow his advice. I knew what I was doing, and he got mad at me. Then I would create little episodes, little situations to get reinforcement for what I wanted to get. At times I would go to the extreme of trying to do exactly what he wanted. I would make myself be the way he wanted me to be. Then I'd change. I'd become indifferent, I'd withdraw from him. I'd play this cat and mouse game. Now what can I do about it?

All this seems to be the patient's last ditch effort to run away.

Doctor: You are playing this cat and mouse game with me, right now.

The therapist at this point decides to make a strong transference confrontation.

Patient: What?

Doctor: The very thing you are describing you did with this fellow you are doing here with me. Right this minute.

Patient: Am I? I must be doing it, then, all the time.

Doctor: Aren't you aware of it?

Patient: No . . . but what shall I do?

Doctor: There you are. How would I know what you should do? Even if I did, do you think I'd tell you?

The therapist makes it clear that he will not support the patient's evading tactics.

Patient: No. It's up to me to find out.

Doctor: Exactly. If so, why do you ask?

Patient: . . . It makes me mad.

Doctor: Now look. We have a golden opportunity, if it is happening between us right now, to examine it and to understand it.

Patient: I can't find out while I am doing it . . . I can't find the reason why I do it. I can't put it in the right perspective. Do you understand? (Becoming tremulous.)

Doctor: Here we go again. You intellectualize again.

Patient (interrupting): I tear myself down. I degrade myself. Are you satisfied? I am defective. Can't you understand? I don't like it this way, but it is the truth. I want people to like me (practically in tears). I am sensitive to criticism. Do you hear? I want people to like me.

Doctor: Yes.

Patient: It is very important. My parents, I felt, did not love me. Why should I love them?

Doctor: Which came first?

Patient: I don't know, except that I feel guilty.

Doctor: But we do know that you excluded your mother.

Patient (angrily): Well, I resented my mother picking on my father all the time. This attitude of hers was not justified at all. She sucked my father into the arguments, and I would get so angry that I would wish my mother would go away and disappear. I wanted to get rid of her. It was her fault. Do you hear? *Her fault.*

Doctor: So you are angry at your mother yet you learned manipulating men from her.

Patient: . . . I never thought of it this way! . . . I never did . . .

Doctor: You also wished your mother to disappear.

Patient: I felt so guilty, because it was like wishing my mother dead.

Doctor: Precisely. This feeling of guilt followed your wish to get rid of your mother. You justified yourself by convincing yourself that your mother did not love you. Being a woman, and having learned your mother's tricks, such as manipulating men, you had no use for her any more, so you had the wish to get rid of your mother . . .

Patient: Oh, my God! . . . I just remembered as you started to speak that I had the thought how nice it would be to live together and have no more fights. (Blushing.)

Doctor: Together, eh?

Patient: The funny thing is that I (smiling broadly) — well, I idolized my father, but my father (giggling) could not fill my expectations, either.

Doctor: Why do you giggle?

Patient (seriously): You touched on something very real. I know it. I had always a wish to have different parents. I have felt guilty about this. You see, my father did not live up to my expectations, either.

Doctor: What expectations?

Patient: I enjoyed doing things together with my father, but many times my brother interfered; I remember my father wanted me to take my brother in a stroller when we were going out for a walk. I hated my brother for that . . . I remember I used to go to my father's office when I was in high school. We were together then. I would bring him his sandwich, and we would eat together. He used to confide to me about his fights with my mother. Can't you see? This is why I wanted to keep them apart. This is why I wanted to get rid of my mother.

The patient's face assumed an exalted expression; and, with much feeling, she added, "During those times I felt so important."

Doctor: For someone who never has any feeling!

Patient (tremulously): Yes . . . but you see it was different earlier when my brother was around. It was then that all my expectations were shattered.

Doctor: And you never forgave your father!

Patient (in tears): I felt what I had to give him was not important. (Weeping.) . . . I felt so angry, so sad . . . so terribly lonely . . . I felt like nothing.

Doctor: Your love for your father, your disappointment in your expectations, your anger at your brother — the thought that he was better, your sorrow and your self-degradation, and finally your loneliness have all been hidden behind this intellectualizing, controlling mask of yours — behind which you hide. Now we can see your true feelings.

Patient (continuing to weep): I know. I know how important all that was.

Doctor: Not "was", *is*, because this is what you do with fellows . . . Let's see how much of this you will remember next time.

This is a classic interview in the height of the treatment. Not only the transference is at full bloom but also the patient is experiencing during the hour all sorts of conflicting emotions: sadness, guilt, anger, joy, exaltation, loneliness. All these feelings are clearly associated to her basic conflict with her parents.

The patient failed to keep her sixth interview. She telephoned at the appointed time to say she was very busy at school and was delayed. I said that we should talk about it all the next time.

Seventh Interview

The patient was five minutes early and came to the office breathlessly.

Doctor: Well!

Patient: You said on the phone "let us talk about it." Well, I didn't forget the last session.

Doctor: Of course, you just wanted two weeks to digest it!

Patient: No. It's awful . . . No! (Speaking quickly, she proceeded to give elaborate details of what had happened at the college which interfered with her being able to keep her last appointment. After a while she slowed down and started to smile.) I see what I am doing! Well, I wanted you to know that it was not that I did not want to come.

Doctor: Is it possible that you didn't?

Patient: It's awful. I feel guilty about it.

Doctor: Guilty? What about it?

Patient: All these feelings about my mother that we talked about, and I kept them alive all this time.

She looked pensive, then she smiled and proceeded at high speed talking about having gone home after Christmas during the past week. She spent much time describing the difficulties with the airlines, the Florida traffic, and so on.

Patient: They think you are crazy when you want to go to Georgia. Everybody says, 'Aren't you going to Florida, dear?' Well, it was my father who helped me make the arrangements. I left the day following the missed appointment. I had planned to talk about it, but then all these complications came up.

Doctor: Hmm.

She continued discussing the details about her reservations.

Doctor: How are things at home?

Patient: Awful . . . I mean . . . you know . . . I felt very guilty about my mother. No one yelled, but there was the usual bickering in the background . . . I felt very guilty about the idea that at one time I wanted my father all to myself and the wish to get rid of my mother, or throw her out of her position — all that stuff you know . . . It was a depressing weekend. (Smiling.) There were some good points, too. My brother was very nice. He read some of the stuff I wrote for college . . . some of my essays . . . he said I was magnificent.

Doctor: Did you enjoy the compliments?

Patient: I felt very guilty; but, of course, I did like them. My parents were also very nice to me. My mother was very nice, yet I felt so bad.

Doctor: Tell me about it.

Patient: Well, . . . you see I was full of feelings this time. It was so different from last summer. It was so different this time.

Doctor: But you said it was awful.

Patient: Well, because of my mother.

Doctor: Of course it is difficult because you love your mother. One does not identify with someone whom one doesn't like.

Patient: Yes. I do. I do love my mother. Actually, you know, I don't like my father in many ways. There are some things he does which annoy me a great deal.

Doctor: I understand. You see the *timing* is of the greatest importance. There are certain feelings which existed at one time and are inappropriate at another time. When all this becomes confused, when these various time levels become mixed up, all sorts of difficulties are likely to come up.

Patient: I start to see that . . . There was this huge thing that happened. My father was in tears. It was all about his wanting to take my brother and me to visit some relatives.

She went into elaborate details about the quarrel between her mother and father, but emphasized that she did not feel detached this time, but actively took her mother's side because she thought her father was unreasonable. She also said that her brother had complimented her, saying that she seemed to have changed a great deal. Then, smiling, she added: "New Year's Eve I went to a party together with my father."

Doctor: You did, did you!

Patient: Oh, it was all very gay . . . Silly, isn't it, to go out on a date with one's father . . . (giggling) . . . but I can assure you I never . . . never had any sexual attraction.

Doctor: Never?

Patient: Well, not after ten or eleven. After I started developing. Actually, really it was after my mother had told me about the facts of life.

She went into detail about having played sexual games when she was eight years old with a little boy who was their neighbor's son. She also described about how, when her aunt was pregnant, she had gone to ask her about how babies were born and questions of that sort. She emphasized her sexual curiosity.

Doctor: We know that there was a time when you walked in

front of your father with no clothes on. How old were you when all this exhibitionism took place?

Patient: Oh, that was much earlier. I know it was before my brother was born . . . Come to think of it, I remember my mother was in the hospital at the time. Maybe it went on . . . No, I do remember my father hugged me a couple of times, but that was all. He didn't seem to like any bodily contact, but my mother was much more affectionate with both of us. Later on in school it was different. All this talk about incest, hell, and punishment, and all that stuff . . . You know something? There was something different this weekend. I felt physical warmth for my brother. It was quite special. There was a closeness between us.

Doctor: Did it have to do with his complimenting you?

Patient: Oh, no, no. It was there as soon as I saw him. I kissed him and gave him a big hug. He is nice, you know.

Doctor: I have no doubt! Anyway, it seems that things are happening.

Patient: You can say that again! I can see things much more clearly, somehow.

Doctor: You seem to.

One may consider that the therapist should have confronted the patient with the acting out of the missed hour. He debated this in his mind but decided that the patient seemed to be aware of what she was doing. Furthermore the details about her visit at home and her behavior with her parents appeared to be just as important. His curiosity was rewarded.

Eighth Interview

The patient was seven minutes late.

Patient: I remember what we talked about last time!

Doctor: Do you want me to compliment you?

Patient: Yes. Oh, no, no, no.

Doctor: You mean yes? Now is it important that you have my approval?

Patient: No . . . well, I mean it must be. This has always been a pattern in me which I do not like in myself, because I pride myself on my own independence.

Doctor: Well, to acknowledge this need in oneself is almost to overcome it. Anyway, what's wrong with wanting to be complimented?

Patient: Yes, I know because this is what happened with my brother as I told you last time. He was nice to me, but it was not all. What came up in the interview about my father and my brother last time was very important. It made much sense. This viewing of my father as a male, and you know I thought about it after the interview. I lumped my father and my brother together, but then I had this attitude about men as "things," which I described to you in the beginning of treatment about my being completely detached with men. That is what I refer to as "thing."

Doctor: I know, yet in this description of yours, you avoid describing the physical attributes of these men.

Patient: You mean whom I consider as a desirable man?

Doctor: Precisely.

Patient: Well it's this "thing" attitude that makes this difficult for me.

She went on like this for a while, but the therapist interrupted her to bring her back to the subject.

Doctor: You are running away.

Patient: . . . You mean the people I find attractive?

Doctor: Whom do you find attractive?

Patient: . . . Someone who is dark, tall, and thin . . . (then adding fast:) They must be well coordinated and athletic. Paul was like that — tall, thin, and then the French fellow was also tall. He was huge.

Doctor: What does your father look like?

Patient (blushing): . . . Well he is tall, thin, and well coordinated, *but* he is not athletic.

Doctor: Oh, I see! (Smiling.)

Patient: I . . . well . . . you know —

Doctor: So in men you look for someone who looks like your father.

Patient: No, all are thin, but all do not have dark hair. Some of the fellows were also athletic. Anyway they have totally different personalities from my father.

Doctor: What does your brother look like?

Patient: He is not very tall, five eleven to be precise, but he is very athletic . . . Oh, well, yes, he is not. What I mean is that both he and mother are very much interested in sports — baseball and stuff like that. My brother, as I told you, is not very well coordinated but he likes sports. He is also very affectionate. He likes physical affection . . . I am repulsed by it . . . What is peculiar, however, is that when I was there after Christmas I felt very relaxed with my brother, as I told you. I also was quite affectionate.

Doctor: What made the difference?

Patient: I don't know.

Doctor: This is a change in you?

Patient (interrupting): Oh, yes . . . I don't know why. You see, my brother does not have any desirable traits. I do not know why it was so different . . . unless, of course, it was the discussion we had here.

Doctor: What do you have in mind?

Patient: Well, the fact that my parents loved me and then when my brother was born I thought that my father did not love me, so I hated my brother and myself after that. Well, what was so different was that I liked my brother this time. After all, it was not his fault.

Doctor: Going back to the subject of your boy friends who have attributes of both your father and your brother. You know, you haven't talked about them very much.

Patient: Well, I go out a lot. The French fellow I met was Catholic, but his attitude about the church was very open.

Doctor: Doesn't he have a name?

Patient: Oh, yeah, I mean his name is Jean Paul. Well, we had a good time together. It was the best relationship I ever had.

Doctor: Was it also a sexual relation?

Patient: Oh, yeah . . . but I gave nothing. I was not a very good sexual partner. I never had an orgasm, and that bothered me a great deal. It was the first time in my life that I had intercourse. After six months I never saw him again. He was wiped out of my memory, as I already told you. He wanted to marry me, but I said no. I considered it for a while but I said no, so he left to go to Lyon in France, then he wrote me a letter. I did not answer, and then more letters started to come. I put them all away. Finally he sent me a telegram and said he will meet me in London and pay for all my expenses, just to have one more talk. He chose London because it was neutral ground between France and the United States. As soon as I decided to go I started to think of marriage, and the more I thought about it the more I thought about my parents' marriage and what a mess that was. I tried to push the thoughts out of my mind. The first few days we had a good time in London, and then I started to find faults with the relationship. I stayed three weeks. He liked me a great deal and wanted to marry me. I had a good time.

Doctor: What happened?

Patient: It was the frigidity . . . you know, I idolized him for six months. Actually the sexual experience changed a great deal for the better. He was aggressive like my father and my brother. He said I was passive in bed. He had vast sexual experience. I was incompetent. I was that big blob of nothing. The next fellow was as inexperienced as I. It was very different. I was domineering both sexually and otherwise. It was he who was passive. I was getting stronger, and it was I who ended the relationship.

Doctor: I thought you did not think of your father and brother as being aggressive.

Patient: In sexual matters I thought they were. I thought that my mother was asexual.

Doctor: Who ended the affair with Jean Paul?

Patient: I did, but it was different. I cried . . . I was weak . . . I was sad. With Danny it was nothing like it, I felt strong.

Doctor: What did Danny look like?

Patient: He liked sports, and he was tall.

Doctor: Oh, I see. He had both your father's and brother's attributes. So you killed two birds with one stone.

Patient (paying no attention): Then I got out a lot after that. I started to go with icky people who were taking acid, you know, LSD trips, drugs, and all that . . . I slept with several guys, and it was very satisfactory, but I felt nothing for them. I could pick and choose anyone I wanted, but I got scared. One day I told myself, "There you are! You go out with all these hippies, all these characters, you sleep with them, you enjoy sex, but where does it all lead? Nowhere. You are getting older. You can't go on like that. You can't spend all your best years like that," and I stopped. Just like that I stopped. And then I met Tim. He was magnificent. Magnificent sexually and otherwise.

Doctor: What happened to that magnificent relationship?

Patient: It ended because of my bizarre behavior. I was too possessive of him. He decided he was not good enough for me. He left me.

Doctor: What about this bizarre behavior?

Patient: Well . . . I can't remember exactly . . . I had all these foolish jealousies. I was not adequate for a magnificent person.

Doctor: But you told me just now that he was not good enough for you and ended the relationship. Who was not good enough for whom, then?

Patient: Well, you see, it was like with my father, when I felt so inadequate that I had nothing at all. But my father paid attention to me after a while. You know I, deep inside, I thought the same thing would happen with Tim. It was a shock when he left me, when he ended it.

Doctor: So you became inadequate just as a way to have your father's attention, to be Daddy's little girl. The question is, does it make you happy?

Patient: Oh, no, no. I hate this feeling. I was so sad after Tim and I separated. I cried and cried.

The rest of the interview was spent recapitulating the early relationship with her father, which already has been discussed in the previous interviews.

The pattern of the patient's heterosexual relations is easily seen as a repetition of the pattern of her relationship with her father. She is able to see it and works hard at it during the hour. It is my impression that this work could not have been done earlier, without the elaborate preparation, the emotional experience, and the clarification of conflicts arising during her childhood, which took place in the last few interviews.

Short-term anxiety-provoking psychotherapy is a systematic, step-by-step process.

Ninth Interview

The patient came five minutes late and was breathless.

Patient: Let me catch my breath . . .

She went on for a while describing the traffic congestion outside the hospital and, then realizing that she was spending too much time on details, said, "Oh, I do remember last week we talked about my relations with men." She then proceeded almost as if narrating a well-studied part of a play, repeating various aspects of the interview of the previous week. Finally, she stopped, was silent for a while, and then said, "Isn't that a good job?"

Doctor: You seem to be looking for my approval again?

Patient: Oh, no, no . . . yes, well you know it shouldn't be this way. I know . . . but it is true I am looking always for other people's reaction. If I detect a reaction in their faces which denotes disapproval or, you know, something like that, I start looking for a fault or flaw or a defect in my argument . . . It is a way of getting what I want or of making sure that all goes well.

Doctor: You seem to be doing all this here with me today. Why is it?

Patient: Well, it doesn't work here. You are not responding. You are not involved in my life, after all. We talk about all these other people. Some of these people are no more involved in it . . .

Doctor: In what way is this a problem? I mean, am I a problem to you?

Patient: You are not a real threat to me. I do not mean that. It is that you are not involved. Yet you are. The involvement is clear yet there is a lack of something.

Doctor: Hm?

Patient: . . . lack of reassurance . . . You are a person — you are human yet you are a sounding board . . . No, no, you are not a sounding board, really, because you say a lot, and sometimes you bring up some very unpleasant things but it is a very "nebulous thing."

Doctor: No. You are hiding in this "nebulous thing." What about —

Patient (interrupting): Well . . . Well, I don't depend on you for love . . . I get all the admiration I want at the school. The other day it bothered me a great deal, because I forgot some details, for the first time. But when I thought about it afterwards, I was pleased because I must be relaxing, somehow. Loosening up . . . (long pause).

Doctor: You seem to be blocked today.

Patient: Really?

Doctor: Maybe not.

Patient: . . . I don't want to talk about my father.

Doctor: Do you dream about your father?

From what follows it is clear that the doctor here pursues a false lead, because he should have continued the subject of the transference, which the patient seems to be willing to talk about.

Patient: No, I don't dream, and if I do I forget them soon afterwards . . .

Doctor: You pause. What are you blocking about?

Patient: . . . Well, you raised the question about dreams, but this is not what I had in mind. Do we have to talk about dreams?

Doctor: No, not at all. You were telling me about your feelings for me.

Belatedly the doctor returns to the issue of the transference.

Patient: I have been disassociating you. I have not let you be important. I do it with other men also. At least I do not get involved with them.

Doctor: What about all this?

Patient: I mean, I do not get involved to the point that the question of marriage comes up. I withdraw, I am not truthful then. I am not faithful. I mean I have no . . .

Doctor: Faithful?

An obvious utilization of the famous slip of the tongue!

Patient: I have no faith in myself.

Doctor: The word faithful implies being faithful to someone else.

Patient: You mean to you? It could —

Doctor: If this is what you mean.

Patient: Well, it has crossed my mind in this way. You know, one must not be interested in anything else outside of psychotherapy. I mean faithful to psychotherapy.

Doctor: Making it faithful to psychotherapy rather than to me takes off the edge of it somehow, but I think it is not really to me that you are faithful but to whom I represent.

Patient: You mean my father.

Doctor: Precisely.

Patient: Well you are tall and thin with dark hair!

Doctor: Hmm, so you thought about it.

Patient: Yes, but I made it into "nebulous thing." I made you a remote kind of figure . . . a sounding board.

Doctor: We know, then, that when you have feelings about men that stir up this association with your father, you make them into things and manipulate them. Do you do this to remain faithful to your father?

Patient: But this terrible feeling comes up immediately. I felt it here already several times.

Doctor: What is this feeling, then?

Patient: Rejection, it's this damned rejection of me as a person . . . It's terrible because I felt my father didn't want me — didn't love me (becoming teary, then her face hardening, wiping her tears irritably) so I say to myself, I'll manipulate you, I'll make you crawl."

Doctor: And that's what you do with your boy friends. You punish them because you are angry at your father for his fictitious rejection of you.

Patient: Fictitious?

Doctor: Yes, it was you who decided that you were ugly, and it was you who felt that you did not like yourself, and it was you who persuaded yourself to blame your father for it, and who proceeded to pretend that he rejected you. The only thing that you told me is that he also liked his son. Isn't a father entitled to love his son?

Patient: Yes, he is. But it is that I do not experience these feelings . . .

Doctor: You were in tears a few minutes ago.

Patient: I know, and I hate myself for it. I don't want to expose myself to you.

Doctor: What is it that you feel so ashamed to show me?

Patient: It's that you may not like me (teary again).

The interview ended on this high note of emotional tension. The patient was greatly relieved and almost ran out of the office.

Again during this hour the therapist moves to clarify the transference, and this tends to help the patient experience her sad feelings of being rejected by her father, as well as her anger. Her wish to manipulate him in order to punish him follows. At this point the therapist thinks that the time has come to confront her with her creation of a fictitious rejection which he supports with the evidence that, on the basis of what she had told him, indeed she had never been rejected by her father. This technical maneuver intensifies the patient's anxiety, which is relieved not by the therapist but by the ending of the hour.

The therapist may be criticized for terminating the interview at such an affect-laden point. What would the patient do? Will she act out as she did in the past by skipping the following hour?

There is a great deal of difference, however, between what is happening during the ninth interview and what transpired during the fifth. The therapist is confident not only that the patient is capable of handling her anxiety well but that she may even be able to utilize it constructively in an effort to understand herself.

Tenth Interview

The patient came on time and started to talk about the tests that she had taken, giving many details about the difficulties she encountered. Then suddenly she exclaimed, "I have changed!"

Doctor: You have?

Patient: Yeah, I feel different — somewhat different. I

thought that several guys I know have changed, and you know they haven't, *I have* . . . I don't view them as machines any more. I have warm feelings.

Doctor: As you had for your brother during Christmas?

Patient: Yes, exactly.

Doctor: Can you give me a specific example about this change in you?

The therapist is very much interested in any tangible evidence of change occurring outside the therapy.

Patient: There is a fellow I have known for a while. Well, I did not like him physically, but I viewed him as a thing, and you know, I was thinking about it. This huge change developed after that interview we had here, and it culminated by my not coming the next time . . . Well, I noticed that I have warm feelings for Jay. I feel very different. We do not have sexual relations, and there is no interest in it at all on my part, but I like him. Well, he reminds me of my father physically. He has an unusual job. He is a nice person. At first I was like a big blob. Nothing. I met him before Christmas. You know, in one of those Christmas parties. Since then we saw each other four or five times . . . You know how it is.

Doctor: No. Now can you give me some details?

Patient: Well, I don't like his attitude about sex. I have a strong feeling of wanting to be idolized as a woman. I think he also has some conflicts in this area, between love and sleeping with people. Well, you see in the beginning — what I mean is that he used to have many views which my father has and I had disagreed with him violently. Now, I don't mind so much. I somehow accept them in a more give and take manner.

She went on giving elaborate details of the various discussions and disagreements with Jay. Having created a situation when Jay had no alternative but to disagree, she interpreted this as a rejection. The parallel with the situation with her father was demonstrated clearly to her.

Patient: You know the thing that made me so happy at the time of the fight was when he called afterwards and apologized.

Doctor: So you won in your battle.

Patient: Yes, but you know the interesting thing is that a somewhat similar situation has developed lately, when *I* called him and *I* apologized. You know, I couldn't believe it at the time when I was doing it. I had never done it before. I kept saying to myself, "You are doing it — you are doing it." I felt so good about it afterwards.

Doctor: There you are. Having relaxed a bit and being able to try a different way of handling the situation, not only you can do it but also you feel good.

Patient: Yes, I know.

The rest of the interview was spent on amplifying and recapitulating the whole issue of her feelings originating at the time she thought her father rejected her when her brother was born and on the ways by which she handled these feelings subsequently in her relations with men.

Eleventh Interview

Patient: . . . I can't think of anything to say . . . I saw Jay and I misinterpreted a statement he made about sex, but it was not as bad as I thought (smiling).

Doctor: Why are you smiling?

Patient: I am happy. I feel much better about my new attitude. I don't feel as closed in. Well, it has something to do with being here . . . I feel it is funny to be so verbal. Well, when I realized so clearly last week during the hour and afterwards how much I manipulated people because of this huge neurosis of mine, I felt depressed about it. I did not like the idea that as a result of these ways of mine I was very alone. I realized that I had rejected everybody . . . Well, I talked to my father.

Doctor: You did!

Patient: Oh, just on the phone. I didn't go to Atlanta. My grandmother died.

Doctor: I am sorry to hear that.

Patient: Well, it was expected. It was very different with my father. I felt much friendlier. When he told me about my grandmother I felt like a little child. I wanted my father to decide for me whether I should go to the funeral or not. This was a change in my attitude.

Doctor: Indeed. From a manipulating powerhouse to a helpless little girl!

Patient: Well, there is such a relief not to feel that I have to manipulate all the time. You know, it takes a lot of effort to keep on doing it.

Doctor: I think that you are more willing to accept yourself as a woman, but you don't have to be a helpless little girl either. Is it necessary to go to extremes?

Patient: Well, no, I can add Jay too . . . I don't manipulate him.

Doctor: And your brother.

Patient: Yes. Well, I made no effort to manipulate anybody except . . .

Doctor: Except?

Patient: I don't know what I meant.

Doctor: What comes to mind?

Patient: . . . I just seemed to be blocked again here.

Doctor: Does it have to do with your talking about pleasant things today?

Patient: I don't know.

Doctor: What comes to mind?

Patient: . . . Impossible.

Doctor: Impossible? Come now.

Patient: My mind is blank.

Doctor: You sound as if it were the first interview today.

Patient: . . . I know it is ridiculous.

Doctor: I did not say that.

Patient: *I* did.

Doctor: You put a value judgment on your attitude.

Patient: I know . . . I guess I do . . . I feel uncomfortable.

Doctor: Well?

Patient: It is ridiculous to tell someone that I like him.

Doctor: So it is a good feeling that you are avoiding.

Patient: Hmm. Hmm.

Doctor: How does it feel inside?

Patient: Wonderful!

Doctor: You know it is just as important to look at the pleasant feelings as it is the unpleasant ones.

Patient: You can't imagine (teary). You can't imagine what a nice feeling it is to be thought well of. My brother thinks I am important. It is so nice to be able to think of positive things about people rather than all these negative things I used to think before . . .

Doctor: You stop again.

Patient: I have such a warm feeling. It is a physical feeling, right now . . . I like it . . . You know what I am trying to say.

Doctor: I know, but you can tell me.

Patient: . . . I feel so good with Jay. We get along so much better, it is in a way similar to the way I feel about my brother. It is so important to be needed, to have something to offer to people.

She continued to talk much more easily about her good feelings for Jay. The therapist was aware that the transference feelings for him have not been discussed adequately and that finally the patient had avoided talking about them, but he thought that if he pushed the issue of the positive transference which was being presented, he would not have heard about all the details of the patient's relation to Jay. It could be argued, of course, that this was a mistake. Anyway, the therapist listened without interrupting her. At the end of the interview he said simply:

Doctor: I think what you said was very important, but you avoided talking about your feelings for me.

Patient: I know, and I feel awful.

Twelfth Interview

Patient (smiling broadly): It was a nice week . . .

The therapist could have used this introductory remark to broach the subject of termination, but he thought that the transference still required further clarification.

Doctor: Hmm.

Patient: No problems at all. Everything was okay . . . The trouble that I have now is not to talk to other men. I get along fine. My trouble has to do with talking to you . . . To you . . .

Doctor: I agree, and this is why I brought it to your attention at the end of last hour. We must overcome this last hurdle, then.

Patient: . . . I feel ill at ease . . . You know, maybe it has something to do with considering psychotherapy as a one-sided conversation . . . and I feel ashamed . . . I feel I am talking to a wall.

Doctor: What do you want me to be like, then?

Patient: Well, I would like you to be easier to talk to; someone with whom one could have a social conversation. Well, you know . . .

Doctor: I don't know.

Patient: . . . Hmm. Well you know, to be more friendly . . . to be a friend of mine . . . Anyway, it is difficult to talk to you.

Doctor: The question is why.

Patient: Yes, I know . . . It is not a question of communication. It is that there is nothing to communicate with . . . a nothing.

Doctor: A "nothing," that is familiar, isn't it?

Patient: . . . Hmm. Yes. It is that there is nothing that I have to offer you.

Doctor: Offer me something . . . nothing . . . what about all this?

Patient: I get irritated at myself.

Doctor: How do you feel?

Patient (with some feeling): Annoyed, irritated. How can I get excited if there is no response, if you don't give me anything. (Blushing.) I feel frustrated.

Doctor: Because I am not your friend?

Patient: Well, no . . . it is this whole nonstructured situation in here. No, it is not that I want you to be a friend; it is something else. It is this atmosphere, this room.

Doctor: What does this remind you of?

Patient: . . . I don't know. I can't put my finger on it . . . (She looked preoccupied and was silent for some time, then she smiled.)

Doctor: You smile.

Patient: Well this being or not being friends business.

Doctor: Yes.

Patient: Well, it is something else . . . You see, I don't need you as a friend . . . This is not what bothers me most. I come in here, and I have nothing to offer you.

Doctor: There we are again "offer me something." We went a full circle and got nowhere. Let me recapitulate. There is this feeling of irritation with me for not responding to you for being a "nonstructured nothing." You say you offer me nothing; you cannot get excited if there is no response. Then there is the atmosphere in this room that reminds you of something . . .

Patient (interrupting): Well if we had something to do. If let's say we could eat a sandwich and talk about baseball or something.

Doctor: You mean like going to your father's office and having lunch together? You "feel so important," you remember?

Patient: I *never* thought of it. I *never* did. Isn't it remarkable!!

Doctor: How did your father react those times?

Patient: Well he was friendly. He complimented me on my clothes. He was very nice. It was then that he used to talk to me about his troubles with my mother. I used to get excited, and I would give him advice and stuff like that.

Doctor: And I don't react in the same way.

Patient: Well, no. You don't respond in the same way. You don't make me feel at ease.

Doctor: This frustrates you. I can see that, but you see my job is not to make you at ease. My job is to help you solve this problem.

Patient: I used to enjoy these visits so much! I felt that I could give something to my father, that he needed me, and this made me feel so good.

Doctor: What intrigues me is your emphasis here on having nothing to offer me. What about that?

Patient: Yes, and this is why the whole thing is confusing, because at these times with my father I felt I had a lot to offer him.

Doctor: But there were other times with your father.

The patient blushed slightly.

Doctor: I think I know what you are thinking.

Patient: You mean?

Doctor: Yes — the times when you were parading in front of your father with no clothes on, when you were exhibiting yourself to him.

Patient (blushing crimson): . . . I had nothing to offer him then, nothing at all . . .

Doctor: So you see how your feelings from two different times in your life were mixed up and expressed in here in reference to me. The episodes with your father in his office occurred when you were fifteen?

Patient: Sixteen and later on.

Doctor: Yes. Of course the time you were running around with no clothes on was at the age of five or so, at the time of your brother's birth.

Patient: Yes, and I remember that it happened after my brother was born.

Doctor: So you can see that these feelings really have nothing to do with me personally. Only this situation has revived feelings that have existed long time ago.

In retrospect one could say that it was worth postponing the discussion of the issue of termination.

The rest of the hour was spent on recapitulating the transference feelings and on reminiscing about various details from her childhood.

Thirteenth Interview

Patient: Well, it was a nice week again. Everything was fine.

Doctor: When shall we stop?

Patient: Stop what?

Doctor: Psychotherapy.

Patient: Well . . . I mean, it's just that everything was fine. I just don't feel that we've solved all the problems.

Doctor: We don't have to solve them all, do we?

Patient: We stopped talking about them. We don't know everything.

Doctor: Maybe we know enough about them.

Patient: But are they going to change? Well, it's one's attitude that continues to change, doesn't it? I mean, that's what I thought.

Doctor: Does it?

Patient: Mine seemed to change — I mean I'm not, I don't seem to be as worried about various things as I was before (long pause) but, uh — (long pause) now I don't think about various things as much as I used to. Uh — I think I've changed in some ways, but I still find myself doing many things in the same way.

Doctor: For instance?

Patient: Well, like, uh, I guess maybe I changed some. I thought, actually (laughing), there was going to be this huge change.

Doctor: No, you couldn't possibly expect to have a huge change in certain things that you have been doing all your life. Lately you function very well, very efficiently. I think you know some of the reasons why you have been, for instance, competing with people. We have talked about your manipulating people such as your mother, friends, people at work, and various young men. It doesn't have to be a huge change. I agree with you that things are going well, and I also expect that your attitudes will continue to change. We don't have to stop right now, but I think we could think about the possibility of terminating treatment.

Patient: Yeah, that's fine. I mean — you know like — see, the main thing is that I don't think about these negative things as much as I did before. Like before it seemed like everything was negative. All I could think about was faults or, you know, the negative side effects. I feel fine about young men, and actually I like discussing these changes in attitude. I don't get neurotic about these things any more.

Doctor: In your opinion, what have we done up to now? How would you recapitulate, let's say, our psychotherapeutic work?

Patient: Well, the reason I came here in the first place had to do with my relations with men. I don't think it was gratifying at all.

Doctor: Hold on just a minute. I wanted to ask in more general terms of your . . .

Patient: Oh, just in the whole thing, oh yes.

Doctor: In terms of your reason for coming which had to do with your unsatisfactory relationships with men . . . has there been a change?

Patient: Yes, there has been a change.

Doctor: So I think the primary reason that brought you to the clinic has been changed. What else did we do?

Patient: Then we discussed my childhood and my relation with my parents and particularly with my father and how I always thought that my parents — my father, in particular, didn't really love me or respect me no matter what I thought. I was trying to be accepted, and all those little things about the fights and how they were all just sort of created so I would be the center of attention. Gaining the attention of my father was important, yet I managed to view my father as sort of a failure as a man, and I decided that anyone in the male role I could manipulate. My feelings about my appearance and how I thought I had nothing to offer after my brother was born, now I understand. I thought I was ugly. I had nothing to offer to people.

Doctor: Now what about this attitude? Do you still feel that this is still true?

Patient: No, no. I feel that I have something to offer people.

Doctor: I think so too.

Patient (laughing): I think the whole thing sort of revolved on these unsatisfactory relationships with men, and it reinforced that feeling of not having anything to offer. I experienced this feeling right here.

Doctor: Yes indeed.

Patient: I do feel much better now.

Doctor: Hmm.

Patient: And then along with that we talked about authority figures; we talked about how I felt about you.

Doctor: And this is something we haven't completed as yet. There was a difficulty in this area last time. Shall we try to understand it today?

Patient: But I, we talked about how I didn't think you were a friend or — didn't act like one.

Doctor: Yes.

Patient: There was also this episode about you in this office and my wish to make it be like having lunch with my father. That was remarkable last week!

Doctor: Hmm.

Patient: I also remember this very funny thing that happened. I don't know if I ever brought it up here before. When I was in class earlier this year it was just ridiculous. There was this guy with whom we used to argue all the time who was just an awful teacher. In fact I even stopped going to his class, I couldn't stand him. Now we never argue in class anymore. He is the supervisor of the students. The whole thing is completely different from the way it was only a few months ago. It's a funny thing, isn't it? There was a change just like that. I now feel that he is capable of giving me lousy grades or something like that if I deserve to get them. I don't think he is a lousy teacher. Come to think of it he is quite good. It is that I used to put him in this position of authority, and I had to rebel against him because I felt I had nothing to offer. Now it has all changed.

Doctor: The same thing happened here. You put me in a position of authority.

Patient: This is what I was thinking. This is why I made the comparison.

Doctor: I think it's a good one.

Patient: Well I — Now even the chairman of the department, I don't feel threatened by him either. We used to disagree a great deal.

She continued to discuss in some detail the problem with the chairman of her department and contrasted it with her present situation, which was peaceful.

Doctor: Since we have been talking about changes in you and since we have been observing these changes in respect to other people, I was wondering what role do you attribute to your psychotherapy in reference to all this?

Patient: You mean in how I communicate with people and things like that?

Doctor: Yes.

Patient: Well, it played a major role. I don't have any problem communicating anymore. I mean I'm not as upset as I was when I came. Well there are still some individuals I don't like, but that is to be expected. I never got along with children in grade school because I never followed their rules; at times I did not do my homework and it was my mother who did it for me if I had some difficulty with it. It was a way to be subversive.

Doctor: When you said that your mother did your home-work if you were having difficulty, in a way she imposed her own standards on your homework. Why did you let her do that?

Patient: Oh, well, Daddy used to do things like that; for example, we'd be going to an amusement park or something and he would say, oh no, you can't wear Bermuda shorts, which is, you know, ridiculous.

Doctor: You did not answer my question, but anyway how did you feel about that?

Patient: I thought it was totally unreasonable, and do you know what I would do, I'd become subversive and I would wear Bermuda shorts under my skirt and he would never know about it.

Doctor: How old were you when all this about Bermuda shorts took place?

Patient: Twelve — No, no I guess it would be older than that because it must have been when I was about sixteen.

Doctor: Now let us try to figure things out about this rebellion. We have established that you had a strong reaction to your brother's birth. After being in a sense the center of attention, things changed, and you became a rebel. From what age? Do you remember? When was the beginning of this?

Patient: Well, it must have been, it must have been the summer when I was five, I was in kindergarten.

Doctor: I see.

Patient: Well, my mother always said that I went two years to nursery school before and that I was very bored with kindergarten because I knew how to do all the things, you know, I knew how to organize all the stuff, see, and when I was in my second year of nursery school I'd always help the teacher hand out stuff, so that apparently when I was in kindergarten I started to do the same thing, which didn't go over well at all. I was too far ahead of the kids in kindergarten.

Doctor: But when was this open rebellion?

Patient: I don't think I openly rebelled.

Doctor: Well, you know what I mean, wearing Bermuda shorts under your skirt. How old were you then?

Patient: Oh, yes, that was very conscious but like when I . . .

Doctor: Now this conscious rebellion, that's what I mean. You said twelve and then sixteen. Could it be that it was at twelve?

Patient: Well, you know (laughing) Dad would never dare to set down the rules of discipline that mother did. I mean, he would occasionally come up with some of these statements all of a sudden if he had a bad day like we weren't to wear Bermuda shorts to the amusement park. I mean, it's just stupid, it's so weird. But mother was very consistent with things like that, you know. Like I needed this one time a date to go to the prom and, oh yes, I had been going out with this fellow, I was only allowed to see him once a week, and so he came over and he had this nice car, it was a convertible and it was a gorgeous day and father said I could go for a ride for one hour. Mother decided that I wouldn't be back by dinner time so she said no, and I was very upset. Then she gave in — she gave in but it was very rare. Usually mother was very consistent on discipline that she handed out. I feel I could get around my father. My brother does the same thing. He knows he can get around my father but not my mother.

She went on at some length talking about her rebellion against her parents and was able to differentiate clearly her reaction to her father's attitude after her brother was born when she was five which was again repeated when she was around twelve. Her rebellion against her mother continued throughout her school years.

Doctor: Well, what about having two more interviews and then we shall terminate?

Patient: Sure, sounds fine.

Doctor: Very good.

Patient: Then I won't have some deep-seated problem to solve before my last visit?

Doctor: It's up to you.

Patient: I always thought I was relatively healthy.

Doctor: I agree. As a matter of fact, I think you are very healthy. I think you had a problem which we were able to examine and then helped you understand it. Your atittude about it has changed. You seem to have loosened up. Your relationships with people seem to have improved markedly. You have done a good job.

Patient: Well, that makes me feel better.

Doctor: Very good. See you next week.

I suspect that the reader may be perplexed and somewhat bored by this interview. He may justifiably ask why the therapist after introducing the subject of termination let the patient ramble on about issues which had been discussed already.

This was done on purpose. It was a way to lessen the shock, and to allow the patient to decide for herself that the idea of termination was a good one.

From the way the patient talks about termination at the end in contrast to the beginning of the hour, it seems clear not only that the therapist was able to minimize the shock but also that the patient seemed to take the whole issue in her stride.

Fourteenth Interview

When I went out to see whether the patient had arrived I saw an attractive young woman sitting down reading a magazine. I thought she was a patient of one of the other psychiatrists. As I returned to my desk I heard a knock on the door, and my patient came in. I had not recognized her. She wore her hair short, was dressed up in a very feminine outfit, and looked like a different person. Smiling she said,

Patient: Everything is fine today. I feel better. (Laughs.) I didn't go to school today.

Doctor: Oh?

Patient: Because I didn't want to — uh — every once in a while I feel sort of queer.

Doctor: What about?

Patient: It was, there was no specific reason why I wasn't going, I just didn't feel like going to school. Like having a special day to do what I wanted to. Well, everything is fine. Now that I know that I don't have to continue coming here I feel fine.

Doctor: But since you brought it up in terms of your feelings about not having to come here anymore, do you think that not going to school is in anyway connected with these feelings?

Patient: Oh, well, you see the only time I didn't go to school is when I felt good — I mean — like it was significant. I haven't done it for about a year. I mean, I, you know, I feel good.

Doctor: This is intriguing!

Patient: Intriguing? Oh, I know — like when I was in the public school and also when I worked during the summer I just couldn't care because we had just ten sick days a year, and I used to take a sick day. But it had absolutely nothing to do with sickness. You know, like all of a sudden I decided that today I was going to write letters, um, that was just great and I wanted to do that right away and not at school. At first I thought, you know, well, I mean like, there was nothing going on at school I was trying to avoid. It was just a drag. And I don't like to lounge around.

Doctor: What did you do today?

Patient: Today I went over to Cambridge and walked around in all the stores and bought things. I know it was a great day, too.

Doctor: So what are you so happy about?

Patient: I don't know. Well, I mean, I feel carefree. I guess I go into those moods. I know things are going along fine in my life. I just feel good I don't usually sit there and ask myself why.

Doctor: But isn't it important to ask oneself — whether one feels happy or not?

Patient: Like, you mean question myself and stuff like that . . .

Doctor: I think it is a good idea to know why one feels the way one does, but since . . . (patient interrupts).

Patient: But you can waste a lot of time doing that.

Doctor: Let's try to figure it out right now.

Patient: You can destroy the feeling if you sit there and think about it all the time.

Doctor: Come now, Miss W., if it can be destroyed so easily then it must be that it is not genuine.

Patient: Oh, okay. Think about it. Eh? (Long pause.) There is no reason, I mean, I really can't think of anything. You know, everything *is* going very well.

Doctor: Can you tell me about that?

Patient: Well, Jay is wonderful. You know, everything is going along fine. So I feel like I am normal. (long pause) Um, now I like Jay and I don't sit there and analyze this anymore — I mean like — hmm (pause) I don't wait for the bad, these sort of awful things to happen. I mean, you know, not being so negative about it.

Doctor: What about Jay?

Patient: What about it? I mean, it's good. You mean just how we get along and stuff like that? Or just anything I want to say? I enjoy being with him, and I guess this is very normal.

Doctor: To like people feels a bit peculiar?

Patient: Right.

Doctor: What about it then?

Patient: I don't know. Well, like when I first started going out with Jay I started condemning all of those people he knows the minute they walked in. It was the same thing with my other dates. I'd talk with them for about five minutes and then I'd make up my mind that I would never go out with them again. As I told you, all this has changed with Jay, particularly after New Year's.

Doctor: You said that you thought our interviews had something to do with it.

Patient: Well, yes, they must have had something to do with my feelings. But it didn't have anything to do with my meeting Jay because it was his sister who fixed me up with him. I can't really pinpoint one real significant thing, you know, other than the interview when I discussed about my parents and . . .

Doctor: What about that?

Patient: About how I felt that they didn't love me?

Doctor: Yes.

Patient: Well, you know, we talked about my looking at people as individuals and not as things, you know, that I can manipulate. I can remember when I first met Jay I thought, "Oh, yecch"! (laughing) and then I thought — you know — I have learned that I must think about people as being individuals, having their own way. I can remember we were talking about something like that at the time. I had never thought about it in this way before. After we demonstrated that there was love, and affectionate feelings about my father and that it was I who felt that I was rejected because he wasn't reacting to me then, you know, from then on Jay suddenly became a different person to me, but before that it was a coincidence. (Doctor interrupts.)

Doctor: But there was another interview. An earlier one when we discussed at length how you felt about the problems of your parents and particularly about your love for your father and your disappointment, your sorrow, and your loneliness? That's the one I . . . (Patient interrupts.)

Patient: Yes, that is the one. I just didn't let people love me anyway. I covered up . . .

Doctor: Let's just recapitulate what happened at that time, because it was a very important interview, following which you did not come. You went home, and you saw things somewhat differently. You came back, and you happened to have met Jay. All this within a short time. Now it is interesting that in a sense, as you said before, you used to pick out people who were peculiar, "icky" was your word. Afterwards you picked someone like Jay and except for one disagreement you changed your attitude. Now both of you are making an effort to get along. Your relationship has been a very good one, and you're very happy. Now I cannot think that all this was coincidence.

Patient: No, I don't think that finding Jay was a

coincidence. I was prepared for it, but the actual meeting . . .

Doctor: I see! Yes, meeting Jay was not the point. It was your attitude about Jay that made the difference. You did not continue to handle him as a "thing." You allowed yourself to see him as a human being.

Patient: No, I never thought that it was a coincidence, but all of a sudden things fell into shape, you know, I learned a lot about myself here. I mean I would have reacted the same way to Jay or anybody else. I could have met someone else, I mean there are millions of people like Jay. Well, there aren't millions of people like Jay, but there are millions of people that represent the same thing that Jay does to me (long pause) things which somehow are tied up with what my parents represent.

Doctor: Uh huh . . . We seem to misunderstand each other today. Do you think it has something to do with termination?

Patient (paying no attention): It all sounds so simple. I mean, I just could never, I don't think I ever realized that before . . . No, there is no misunderstanding.

Doctor: Can you tell me what these things represent now?

Patient: Well, number one, the church. Put that right at the top of the list. (Laughing.)

Doctor: How do you feel about it now?

Patient: What? The church? Well, I mean it's sort of like one of those . . . no! In fact it isn't. My main gripe against the hypocrites is that they sort of control human beings, you know, kind of bring children up so that they are like anybody else, mass produce them all alike, turn them into sort of inhuman beings — removing something from them which is human, making people conform, make them into "things." And I never thought about it . . . lately I began to think about it, and the more I think about it the less I believe in the church. I learned to question my attitudes here. It's my psychotherapy that taught me, you know, to ask questions. As a result I changed. I like men as human beings, but I still don't like the church. It is absolutely ludicrous! But Jay, you know —

Doctor: Now, just a minute. Does Jay think that the whole thing is ludicrous?

Patient: No, I don't think so. No, these were just some things I thought over myself. You see I had built it up to such a degree. My parents and Jay are entitled to their own ideas about church even if I disagree — when I disagreed with my parents I tried to manipulate them. Now I disagree, but I don't want to manipulate anyone any more. It's okay I suppose, to like the church. It is I who do not. I disagree but . . .

Doctor: Yes . . .

Patient: I truly think they're great, all three of them.

Doctor: Yes, but you said that your attitude has changed — not only about people but also about certain things that Jay and your parents represent.

Patient: Oh, but the attitude about the church isn't one of them.

Doctor: But why did you give me the church as an example? That is what I am wondering. What are these things that your attitudes have changed about?

Patient: Oh, you want to know what my attitude has changed about!

Doctor: As I said before we seem to misunderstand each other today.

Patient: Well, maybe . . . I'll give you an example . . . sort of this middle-class type of thing that I've always thought was just awful. Like everybody being so concerned about their cars and all that stuff. I felt so superior to all these people, now somehow I don't make so much of all this. Well I thought it was very significant that I got my hair cut.

Doctor: I was wondering about that!

Patient: What? Yes, I had it cut.

Doctor: I can see. I can see. (Laughing.)

Patient: Um.

Doctor: What made you have it cut?

Patient: Well, first of all, my mother was trying to get me to get my hair cut. And so, you know, I kept it longer. And also it was something like the people I used to know in Cambridge, they were connected with that whole thing. These people were completely removed from anything that was middle class. I didn't like them, really . . .

Doctor: How did the thought occur to you that you should have your hair cut?

Patient: Well, first of all, there is this girl friend of mine who thought that — oh, a long time ago — every once in a while she would suggest that I should cut my hair. I'd get, like thirty thousand calls, and I would say no. Well I thought it was very significant because I was getting a certain amount of attention. Then, Judy, one day we were talking, and she said something about my hair and I thought maybe I would change the color, but I didn't do it. I remember when my mother came to visit me she said the same thing. When I was home at Christmas time, there was absolutely no mention made about my hair, except that I wore it up all the time, and the one particular reference made was that I didn't wear it down. Nobody was too concerned about my hair or anything else and so, you know, I thought it was not very effective — I mean I wasn't getting some kind of attention. Dad just didn't say anything, and then once later on Daddy said, well you know, "Maybe you'd look pretty with your hair cut." I thought maybe I would. Today I just went to this great place on Newbury Street, and I had a great time. I met another friend of mine who had her hair done at the same place and we sort of went together and it was fun, so I had it cut off. I wasn't really going to have it all cut off, I was going to have it trimmed, and then I sort of changed my mind.

Doctor: Are you pleased with it?

Patient: Oh, I love it!

Doctor: Do you think it looks good?

Patient: I got the color changed too. That was last week. Last Saturday. I also decided that I'm going to go to the beauty parlor every Saturday. I thought it was a great idea, I still do.

Doctor: Do you remember we talked about appearances and

your ideas about the way you look? In what way is your cutting your hair related to that?

Patient: Oh, I'm sure it does. I'm more relaxed about myself. Jay thinks I'm magnificent. He thinks I'm beautiful, and so what's the difference whether my hair is short or long?

Doctor: But the question is what do *you* think about yourself?

Patient: Well, I um, my concept of myself has improved one hundred percent.

Doctor: Uh. Mind you, not that I'm in any way saying that the fact that Jay also thinks that you look . . . (Patient interrupts.)

Patient: Oh, but I think that's important.

Doctor: I think it is very important, but what is even more important as far as I'm concerned is that *you* feel one hundred percent better about yourself.

Patient: Yes, I know I feel like I'm just better, that's all.

Doctor: I think you are too.

Patient: Well, I mean the whole idea, the whole thing is fantastic. I decided that my own appearance was sort of yecch. I actually tried to convince myself consciously. I tried to make myself look uglier than I really was. If my mother had said, "Now please look at it rationally; you look better with your hair short" — I mean, at that time I would have been repulsed at the very thought of her interfering. I *had* to be ugly.

Doctor: I think you exaggerated. You emphasized a bit too much how ugly you were and how tall you were. You talked a lot about this during the beginning of psychotherapy. You know, all about having to kneel because you were so tall, when that picture was taken and so on . . . (Patient interrupts.)

Patient: Oh *yes*, I remember that.

Doctor: You used strong words to describe your feelings. The question is, why were you exaggerating? Why did you feel that you had to make yourself ugly? Obviously there was a reason. Why do you think that you wanted to be ugly? Why is it that you viewed your brother as being absolutely angelic, "magnificent" was the word, while you viewed yourself as completely the opposite. Why did you have to continue this attitude up to very recently to make yourself, as you say, look worse. Why?

Patient: Well, all I can remember, as I said before were these pictures of myself and my brother together. My brother was just a gorgeous child . . . (Doctor interrupts.)

Doctor: Yes you told me about that.

Patient: I don't understand why, exactly, I seem to remember these pictures vividly. Unless of course I thought that my parents thought that my brother was gorgeous or something.

Doctor: Hmm.

Patient: Yet I don't remember anything being said about that at all. All I can remember is that I associate it with the time my brother was younger.

Doctor: Yes. Now if your brother was gorgeous, why did you have to be the opposite?

Patient: I don't know — because I didn't want to compete — do you think? I don't know why I wanted to be ugly, because obviously that wasn't going to get any attention. I don't think I consciously thought of myself as being ugly or oversized when I was age six.

Doctor: Indeed! So what about your parents . . . (Patient interrupts.)

Patient: My brother was a new baby.

Doctor: Yes, what did that make you feel like?

Patient: It made me feel that I was not with the rest of the group.

Doctor: Yes.

Patient: Therefore there was some reason why I was being rejected, right?

Doctor: Hmm.

Patient: And so I interpreted it; I blamed the rejection on being ugly.

Doctor: Um — well . . . Yes, but we know that . . .

Patient: Or not wanted?

Doctor: Why?

Patient: Because my brother had taken over being the center of attention. I guess I thought it must be because I was an ugly girl.

Doctor: Yes, and your brother was . . .

Patient: He was a boy!

Doctor: Ah, ha! You see, not "ugly girl," just simply a *girl!*

Patient: Oh, I see! Would it be different if he was a girl?

Doctor: Oh come on now! Let's not speculate on what would have been. Perhaps. Who knows? But you are, even now, so resistant to see something that it so simple.

Patient: But, it's too simple. It's simple, it really is!!

Doctor: Well, it's too simple, I agree with you; but that's why you had a problem. You thought you were rejected because you were a girl. There was something . . .

Patient: I mean it seems so much more simple than anything else, you know.

Doctor: Of course it is. It's very simple. It meant being a girl was no good. But you didn't like that so you invented the word "ugly" to put in front of the word girl.

Patient: Oh, I went through all kinds of stages when I tried to identify with boys.

Doctor: We know what happened when other people were admiring you? When they were interested in you as a woman. Jean Paul . . .

Patient: Yes.

Doctor: Jean Paul and various other young men and you were absolutely convinced that . . . (Patient interrupts.)

Patient: I just thought of them as merely "a thing," because I had nothing.

Doctor: Uh huh. There you are!

Patient: Well, because I can remember going through all kinds of stages — being a tomboy and stuff like that — and this was exactly the way I was even up to now. The whole thing, you know, completely permeated my life. I tried — I pretended I had to be a boy.

Doctor: All your life until you finally came here and had a chance to examine your life. It wasn't clear because even up to this minute you avoided those feelings. We spent three hours here talking about your being rejected, about how ugly you are, emphasizing your own ugliness, emphasizing the angelic qualities of your brother, but you never connected the two. You never thought to look at yourself. Take a look at yourself. It's very simple. If your father had neglected you as you said he did, or rejected you as you thought he did, it must have been for a reason. You concluded a little too easily that the reason why he rejected you was because your brother was so handsome and you were so ugly. You did not consider another and much simpler reason; namely, that you were a girl and he was a boy. This did not come up until now.

Patient: Of course!

Doctor: Yes. (Laughing.)

Patient: That never occurred to me at all. It just simply didn't. The whole thing is just a complete shock, I mean, you know!

Doctor: Yes. You see how the intellect cannot compete with the feelings.

Patient: Actually cover it all up with all this stuff?

Doctor: Yes.

Patient: Really?

Doctor: Well, you tried to. I'm very impressed by this genuine surprise. You are so used to rationalizing in all these ways, as you did in the beginning of the hour today, that the whole thing becomes a total surprise, even if it is so simple. Now did anything else happen?

Patient: Oh, the whole thing comes to me now . . . it's all sort of like going around. I know for one thing I always got along with men a lot better than I get along with women. Yet it was very funny, it was not like a male-female relationship, like the one I have with Jay now. It has always been very different. I had some very good friends that are men, but they never saw me as being a woman. Those who did I manipulated or I rejected. I was also rejecting the notion of being a woman, period. I was trying to turn into a sort of "thing," that had nothing to offer.

Doctor: Yes. An intellectual nothing!

Patient: I can see what you mean by this intellectual nothing. You see, like all along that we've been discussing this problem,

I just told myself that I did not believe it. The first time it became meaningful was when we talked about Dad's rejection. Obviously it is true.

Doctor: Well, it is true, because for the first time you talk like a woman. And you look like one.

Patient (laughing): But I am one.

Doctor: Well of course you are! But you've been hiding it.

Patient: But don't you think that actually all along I was coming to this conclusion.

Doctor: Of course you were.

Patient: Because like even as far back as last Christmas I felt much different.

Doctor: I know.

Patient: On occasions, not with Jay, but with other men, at school I still feel this other kind of attitude, and there is such difference between the two!

Doctor: Well, it takes time to learn to adjust to your new attitude. Actually there is nothing unusual, really. I think that you were a perfectly feminine little girl except that you concluded that you lacked something, that there was something wrong with you when your brother was born, after you saw all the excitement. So you started . . .

Patient: It's really funny. I mean that a little thing like that influenced my whole life. It's true I can see the whole thing happening. Obviously I was jealous of the boy because I wanted to be one too. You know, I think it is very important. It's really amazing!! It's awful hard work, but all the things that we talked about before become so clear now. I really couldn't see what kind of conclusion we were coming to . . . outside this second. I feel so much better. I wasn't dwelling on all of these things today, but the minute I came in here you started to press me to talk about all this stuff.

Doctor: You told me that you wanted me not to push you in this area. Even today you did not want to question why you felt so good because this feeling might go away. You wanted me to ask you inconsequential questions. When I didn't conform you got angry. Well, that was resistance!

Patient: Oh, because you weren't directing the questions?

Doctor: Yes. After all you had nothing to offer, nothing to give. It was the same thing in psychotherapy here with me, as with everybody else since that early time. You had to be told what to do. I had to give you permission, advice, and so forth. In this way you could manipulate and control me as you did the others. Although you did not like it, you had the courage to examine your relationship with me. Once you did this and understood that it repeated the old patterns there was no problem left. When you talked about your feelings about me as a person, not as some kind of equipment or "thing," it was the beginning of the end of this old attitude.

Patient: Well I don't know exactly why I did such rotten things, but I can still see myself doing them. In other words, I still have the urge to manipulate in order to obtain some goal, irrespective of whether it is beneficial or negative.

Doctor: Do you think you're going to continue to do that after today?

Patient: Not with everybody. No.

Doctor: I don't think so, either. You understand yourself. You have become human and feminine again. And you are relaxed because you worked hard during psychotherapy. But why waste all your time and abilities in doing things that are entirely unnecessary? The urge may still persist for awhile, but if you continue in the future trying to utilize what you learned in here, if you continue to remember why you had to manipulate people and why you had to deny your femininity, then I am sure you will be able to solve any problem you may have to face in the future.

Patient: Well, I'm much more relaxed. I was very upset when I was trying to manipulate people. I did not like it at all.

Doctor: I'll see you in two weeks for our last interview.

Patient: Okay.

Although the therapist was convinced that the main job of the therapy had been accomplished, he was surprised to see such a startling change in the patient's appearance. It was because of this that he decided to investigate the area of the patient's ideas about her body image, although he thought that the subject was much too complex to be dealt with in short-term psychotherapy. From what ensued, he was gratified that this issue was also dealt with and clarified, even if it happened at the expense of discussing the feelings regarding termination of the treatment.

Fifteenth and Final Interview

The patient came in beaming.

Patient: Everything is going very well. (She smiled broadly.)

Doctor: Fine.

Patient: I am aware that this is our last interview . . . you got a new head. What is it?

Doctor: What do you mean?

Patient: This bust over there. Is it on public display?

Doctor: Oh I see. Well it is the sculpture of one of my professors. I don't know what you mean "on public display." Do you like it?

Patient: Well, yes. He must have been very handsome.

Doctor: He still is. He is also a famous scientist, a great teacher, and a fine man.

Patient: What is his name?

Doctor: Dr. Stanley Cobb.

Patient: Oh, I see . . . Well I have been working hard the past two weeks, and I solved a new problem that had developed at school. (She then proceeded to describe in detail how she was able to help a girl friend of hers who was in trouble with one of the professors, by listening to her feelings without trying to tell her what to do and control her. She went on like this for a while, then suddenly she stopped.) "I thought a great deal about this being our last hour."

Doctor: Well, what about?

Patient: I was very excited when I left here last time. I felt good. I felt as if a great load had been lifted. The main thing that pleases me most is that I don't have the need to think rationally all the time, as I used to do. Also, my attitude for Jay seems to have changed.

Doctor: Oh?

Patient: Well yes. You know. I can assess the situation more realistically. I do not want to rush into any marriage, now that

I have found my freedom. I like Jay, but I am not so wildly enthusiastic as I felt a few weeks ago. I seem to be more settled, more down to earth. I felt and I feel good . . . very good.

Doctor: What are your plans for the future?

Patient: I would like to go to Europe. I don't have a well-defined plan, but it would be nice to go and spend the whole summer. Maybe stay there. It would be nice.

Doctor: See Jean Paul?

Patient: Oh! No. No. All that is finished.

Doctor: Any other plans?

Patient: Well, yes. I mean no. I want to get married and have a family but not right away. I want some time to think things out. This treatment was so concentrated, so much happened in these few weeks. I need some time to sort things out. All the pieces are there, and I know how to put them together. I don't know yet about marriage, but I do want to get married some time. I don't see marrying Jay. Another thing that I have been thinking about lately is that I am not as dependent as I was. I used to be over-dependent, particularly on these guys I used to go out with in the past, and as a reaction I felt the need to control them. All this is very different now. The need now is to be alone for a while. I like myself better.

Doctor: Hmm.

Patient (enthusiastically): Without *any* doubt in my mind, this is due to psychotherapy, and it makes me feel great. I don't think any more about how ugly I look. I used to all the time. As I said, as a matter of fact, I don't think I look so bad at all!

Doctor: I am glad to hear it.

Patient: Well, I try to find out why I think and I do what I do. I plan to continue doing this in the future. This gives me security . . . I feel healthy. I also feel a bit sad.

Doctor: So you think that we have done a good job here. I agree. You also feel you understand yourself better and are more relaxed. It is understandable that you feel a little sad. Endings are always sad. I feel a little sad myself.

Patient: Really? I am glad. We *have* done a good job.

Doctor: Well I think it is a good idea to stop. (They shook hands.)

Follow-up

The patient was interviewed by an independent evaluator who saw her three months after the end of her treatment in a follow-up interview. This is what he had to say: "She sees herself as vastly improved. She states that she is able to do things now which she had been unable to do before, that she is less afraid of relating than she previously was, and that she has understood a number of relationships which have previously interfered with her life."

He also thought that she still suffered from her separation from her therapist, for whom her positive feelings still existed. He concluded, "She is therefore improved and seems headed in a direction where she can have some insight. She seems to have learned the model of self evaluation."

A questionnaire was sent to the patient eight months later. Here is what she had to say at that time:

I have a much more positive attitude about myself and about my feelings for other people. I feel I can respond more to an emotional climate than before. I can feel in a deeper way. I have much greater insight into what my feelings were and are for my parents, and this has helped me respond differently to those around me, and particularly to men. I am better able to respond to the way I feel about men in a relationship because of the insights obtained about my father and mother.

Sometimes it is hard always to think about what is "therapeutic" and then to act. I have done a lot more problem-solving since I terminated therapy. I don't think I was ready to fully accept some of the things discussed during the therapy sessions at that time. I have not only been able to reason things out, but also to feel emotionally and respond.

She answered also that her symptoms still existed "to some

extent," that she felt "much better than [she] ever had before" about herself, and that she was able to utilize what she learned during this treatment. She answered that she had developed considerable self-understanding and that therapy continued to have an effect on her. Her attitude about what she said and did seemed to have changed. All in all, she seemed satisfied with herself and felt no need for further treatment. One year later another questionnaire was sent, but it was returned. She had departed from Boston and left no address.

One may anticipate some criticism at this point. Only the successful cases have been chosen for this book! What happens to all the failures? This would be justified criticism if the intent had been to present case reports as "cures." This is not what I had in mind. There are several cases which I would consider as failures, but as such they could not have been used to demonstrate adequately the techniques of short-term anxiety-provoking psychotherapy. Since this was my primary purpose for presenting the clinical material I have chosen these particular reports as representative of what was done.

The results obtained by this kind of short-term psychotherapy demonstrate quite adequately that this treatment is no panacea, but rather a fairly useful technique, which, it is hoped, will be added to our therapeutic armamentarium. Short-term anxiety-provoking psychotherapy encourages patients to make their own choices and teaches them how to free themselves from their neurotic chains and how to become and remain independent. This in my opinion is the crucial point.

NOTES AND INDEX

NOTES

Preface

1. William Blake, "Auguries of Innocence," in *Poetry and Prose of William Blake*, ed. Geoffrey Keynes (London, the Nonesuch Press, 1932), p. 118.

Introduction

1. P. E. Sifneos, "Reflections on the Education of the Psychiatrist," in *Psychotherapy and Psychosomatics* (Basel, S. Karger, 1967), pp. 260-272; "Psychodynamics and Psychotherapy," in *Nordisk Psykiatrisk Tidsskrift*, 24 (1970), 116-129.

1. The First Patient

1. This case appeared in shorter version in : P. E. Sifneos, "Phobic Patient with Dyspnea: Short-Term Psychotherapy," *American Practitioner and Digest of Treatment*, 9 (June 1958), 947-953.

2. Psychological Process as a Dynamic Continuum

1. L. Pauling, "Orthomolecular Psychiatry," *Science*, 160 (April 19, 1968), 265.
2. R. R. Grinker, "An Essay on Schizophrenia and Science," *Archives of General Psychiatry*, 20 (January 1969), 1-25.
3. G. P. Sachett, "The Persistence of Abnormal Behavior in Monkeys following "Isolation Rearing," in *The Role of Learning in Psychotherapy*, ed. Ruth Porter (London, J. and A. Churchill, 1968), pp. 3-26.

4. N. E. Miller, "Visceral Learning and Other Additional Facts Potentially Applicable to Psychotherapy," in *The Role of Learning in Psychotherapy*, pp. 295-309.

5. P. E. Sifneos, "Manipulative Suicide," *Psychiatric Quarterly*, 40 (July 1966), 525-538.

3. A Concept of Emotional Crisis

Certain parts of this chapter have appeared in: P. E. Sifneos, "A Concept of Emotional Crisis," *Mental Hygiene*, 44 (April 1960) 169-180.

1. P. E. Sifneos, C. Gore, and A. Sifneos, "A Preliminary Psychiatric Study of Attempted Suicide as Seen in a General Hospital," *American Journal of Psychiatry*, 112 (May 1956), 883-889.

2. H. C. Schulberg and A. Shelton, "The Probability of Crisis and Strategies for Preventive Intervention," *Archives of General Psychiatry*, 18 (May 1968), 553-559.

4. Two Different Kinds of Therapy of Short Duration

Certain parts of this chapter have appeared in my papers: P. E. Sifneos, "Two Different Kinds of Psychotherapy of Short Duration," *American Journal of Psychiatry*, 123 (March 1967), 1069-1074 (copyright 1967 by the American Psychiatric Association); "Short-Term Anxiety-Provoking Psychotherapy: An Emotional Problem-Solving Technique," *Seminars in Psychiatry*, 1 (November 1969), 389-399.

1. P. E. Sifneos, *Ascent from Chaos: A Psychosomatic Case Study* (Cambridge, Mass., Harvard University Press, 1964).

5. Crisis Intervention

1. P. E. Sifneos, "Crisis Psychotherapy," in *Current Psychiatric Therapies*, ed. J. Masserman (New York, London, Grune and Stratton, 1966), pp. 125-128.

2. C. G. Gross, Review of *Integrative Ability of the Brain* by I. Konorski, *Science*, 160 (May 10, 1968), 652-654.

3. P. E. Sifneos, "Preventive Psychiatric Work with Mothers," *Mental Hygiene*, 43 (April 1959), 230-236.

6. Selection of Patients

Parts of this chapter have appeared in: P. E. Sifneos, "The Motivational Process: A Selection and Prognostic Criterion for Psychotherapy of Short Duration, *Psychiatric Quarterly*, 42 (April 1968), 271-279, and

"Two Different Kinds of Psychotherapy of Short Duration," *American Journal of Psychiatry*, 123 (March 1967), 1069-1074 (copyright 1967, the American Psychiatric Association).

1. P. E. Sifneos, "The Interdisciplinary Team," *The Psychiatric Quarterly*, 43 (January 1969), 123-130.

2. P. E. Sifneos, "Short-Term Anxiety-Provoking Psychotherapy," *Seminars in Psychiatry*, 1 (November 1969), 389-399.

3. P. E. Sifneos, "Clinical Observations on Patients Suffering from a Variety of Psychosomatic Illnesses," the Seventh European Congress of Psychosomatic Medicine, *Acta Medica Psychosomatica* (Rome, 1967), pp. 452-459.

4. P. E. Sifneos, *Ascent from Chaos: A Psychosomatic Case Study* (Cambridge, Mass., Harvard University Press, 1964).

5. D. Rapaport, *On the Psychoanalytic Theory of Motivation*, Nebraska Symposium on Motivation (Lincoln, Neb., University of Nebraska Press, 1960); R. S. Peters, *A Concept of Motivation* (New York, Humanities Press, 1959); K. B. Madsen, Theories of Motivation. *A Comparative Study of Modern Theories of Motivation* (Copenhagen, Denmark, Munksgaard, 1961); J. D. Frank, "Individual Differences in Certain Aspects of the Level of Aspiration," *American Journal of Psychology*, 10 (1954).

6. S. Silverman, "The Role of Motivation in Psychotherapeutic Treatment," *American Journal of Psychotherapy*, 28 (April 1964), 212-229.

7. S. Rado, "On Motivation," *Short-Term Psychotherapy*, ed. L. Wolberg (New York, Grune and Stratton, 1965), pp. 67-84.

8. P. E. Sifneos, L'utilisation par un peintre de ses rêves et de ses fantasmes au bénéfice de son activité créatrice, *Revue française de psychanalyse*, 27 (July 1964), 591-608.

9. J. P. Sartre, *The Words* (New York, Braziller, 1964), pp. 113 and 148.

7. Technique

Parts of this chapter have appeared in: P. E. Sifneos, "Psychoanalytically Oriented Short-Term Dynamic or Anxiety-Provoking Psychotherapy for Mild Obsessional Neuroses," *Psychiatric Quarterly*, 40 (April 1966), 271-282.

1. M. T. McGuire, *American Journal of Psychotherapy*, 22 (April 1968) 218-232. M. T. McGuire and P. E. Sifneos, "Problem-Solving in Psychotherapy," *Psychiatric Quarterly*, 44 (October 1970), 667-674.

2. J. S. Bruner, *On Knowing: Essays for the Left Hand* (Cambridge, Mass., Harvard University Press, 1962); Toward a Theory of Instruction (Cambridge, Mass., Harvard University Press, 1966).

3. P. E. Sifneos, "Short-Term Anxiety-Provoking Psychotherapy," *Seminars in Psychiatry*, 1 (November 1969), 389-399.

4. D. H. Malan, *A Study in Brief Psychotherapy* (Springfield, Ill., Charles C. Thomas, 1963) and *The British Journal of Medical Psychology*, 32 (1959), 86-105.

5. P. E. Sifneos, "Dynamic Psychotherapy in a Psychiatric Clinic," in *Current Psychiatric Therapies*, ed. J. Masserman (New York, Grune and Stratton, 1961), pp. 168-174.

6. S. Freud, "The Dynamics of Transference. On Transference Love on Beginning Treatment," in *The Complete Psychological Works of Sigmund Freud*, vol. XII (London, Hogarth Press, 1958).

7. E. Glover, *The Technique of Psychoanalysis* (New York, International Universities Press, 1955).

8. R. Greenson, *The Technique and Practice of Psychoanalysis* (New York, International Universities Press, 1967).

9. F. Alexander and T. French, *Psychoanalytic Psychotherapy* (New York, Norton, 1945).

10. F. Deutsch and W. Murphy, *The Clinical Interview*, vol. I (New York, International Universities Press, 1954).

11. R. Knight and C. Fredman, *Psychoanalytic Psychiatry and Psychology* (New York, International Universities Press, 1954).

12. E. V. Semrad et al., "Brief Psychotherapy," *American Journal of Psychotherapy*, 20 (October 1966), 576-599.

13. P. E. Sifneos, "Learning to Solve Emotional Problems: A Controlled Study of Short-Term Anxiety-Provoking Psychotherapy," in *The Role of Learning in Psychotherapy*, ed. Ruth Porter (London, J. and A. Churchill, 1968), pp. 87-97.

14. H. Strupp, "Teaching and Learning in Psychotherapy," *Archives of General Psychiatry*, 21 (August 1969), 203-212.

15. O. Fenichel, *Psychoanalytic Theory of Neurosis* (New York, Norton, 1945).

8. Results

1. P. E. Sifneos, "Dynamic Psychotherapy in a Clinic," in *Current Psychiatric Therapies* (New York, Grune and Stratton, 1961), pp. 168-174.

2. P. E. Sifneos, "Seven Years' Experience with Short-Term Dynamic Psychotherapy," in *Selected Lectures*, 6th International Congress of Psychotherapy, London, 1964 (New York, S. Karger, 1965).

3. D. H. Malan, *A Study of Brief Psychotherapy* (London, Tavistock, 1963).

4. P. E. Sifneos, "Learning to Solve Emotional Problems: A Controlled Study of Short-Term Anxiety-Provoking Psychotherapy," in *The Role of Learning in Psychotherapy*, ed. Ruth Porter (London, J. and A. Churchill, 1968), pp. 87-97.

5. P. E. Sifneos, "Effects of a Short-Term Psychiatry Course on the Attitudes of Medical Students and Their Teachers," *Psychiatric Quarterly*, 4 (1968), 639-646.

6. D. H. Malan, *A Study of Brief Psychotherapy*; "On Assessing the Results of Psychotherapy," *British Journal of Medical Psychology*, 32 (1959), 85-105; Malan, et al., "A Study of Psychodynamic Changes in Untreated Neurotic Patients," *British Journal of Psychiatry*, 114 (1968), 525-551.

INDEX

Agoraphobia, anxiety and, 147–168
Alexander, F., 107, 115, 116, 120
Anxiety, 24, 27, 35, 57, 83, 194,
  213; factors leading to, 33–43;
  normal versus excessive, 24–25,
  35, 78; with paranoid ideas, 55.
  See also Agoraphobia, anxiety and;
  Examination phobia, anxiety and;
  Heterosexual difficulties, anxiety
  and; Homosexuality, anxiety and;
  Psychotherapy, short-term anxiety-
  provoking; Psychotherapy, brief
  anxiety-suppressive; Psychotherapy, long-term anxiety-suppressive
Autoktonism, 93, 116, 120, 201

Behavior, 22, 33, 46, 50, 56; evaluation of maladaptive, 22, 28, 57–
  59; and genetic factors versus
  environmental factors, 22–23;
  strengths, 44, 70, 83, 112, 142;
  structure, 27, 46, 59
Beth Israel Hospital, 141
Biochemical pathology, 3–4
Boston, 76, 138, 141, 288
Brain function, 3, 22, 64, 95
Bruner, J., 95

Chromosomes, Y, 22
Clarification, 7, 98, 99, 115, 143,
  219; of conflicts, 256; as technical
  tool, 113
Cobb, S., 285

Colitis, ulcerative, 82
Community mental health, 1–2, 4–5,
  25–27, 32–37
Confrontation, *see* Therapist-patient
  relationship, confrontation
Crisis, *see* Emotional crisis
Curiosity, 86, 88, 89, 90, 94, 118,
  120, 251

Defense mechanisms, 21, 33, 35, 42,
  54, 61, 84; adaptive, 129, 137;
  and anxiety, 35; counterphobic,
  21; denial, 54; displacement, 21,
  84, 107, 137, 167; distortion, 54;
  introjection, 61; isolation, 84;
  maladaptive, 137; new, 129;
  pathological, 61. *See also* Projection
Dependence, 99, 115
Depression, 31, 130, 134
Deutsch, F., 109
Diagnosis, 43, 75–92 passim, 101,
  149, 198

Emotion, 4, 32, 35, 42, 71, 80–81,
  99, 108, 112, 114, 116, 121, 158,
  159, 193, 198, 212, 248
Emotional crises, case studies, 30,
  36–37, 38–39, 39–40; definition
  of, 29; evaluation of intensity, 57–
  60; factors in, 32–33; and intervention case studies, 59–61, 63,
  65–66, 67–69, 69–71; and painful
  state, 33–36; and prevention of

neurosis, 41–42, 64–71; role of drugs in, 48; role of environmental resources in, 48

Environment, attempt to manipulate, 36–37; hostile, 84; rearrangements in, 127; role of, 22, 23

Evaluation, *see* Patients, diagnosis of; Psychotherapy, diagnosis of type needed; Psychotherapy, short-term anxiety-provoking, criteria for selection of patients

Examination phobia, anxiety and, 194–213

Existential philosophy, developments in, 2

Factors in emotional illness, biochemical, 44; biological, 2; environmental, 22, 23, 44, 84; fantasy, 4, 5, 55, 81, 87, 89, 90, 97, 108; genetic, 22, 44; precipitating, 15

Feelings, 34, 54, 81, 82, 125, 213, 232, 261; access to, 80, 171; ambivalent, 108, 121; angry, 66; of annoyance, 130; of antagonism, 172; associated with basic conflict, 248; description of, 14; during interview, 80, 115, 118, 236; evading of, 224; from past, 108; from present, 108; guilt, 149; hostile, 55; jealous, 184; negative, 115, 118; painful, 33, 34, 88, 90, 105, 108; paradoxical, 178; pleasurable, 88; positive, 56, 80, 100, 105, 108, 115, 118, 125, 129, 135, 168, 287; regarding termination, 212, 285; sad, 259; as source of motivation, 88; unpleasant, 117; ways to deal with, 259; about women, 175

Fenichel, O., 121

Flexibility, 83, 88, 94, 171; as selection criterion for short-term anxiety-provoking psychotherapy, 80, 82

French, R., 107

Freud, S., 2, 107, 109, 120

Frigidity, anxiety and, 147–168

Genetics, developments in, 2, 22–23

Glover, R., 107, 108, 121

Greenson, R., 107

Gross, C., 64

Harvard University medical students, 77

Health, *see* Community mental health

Heterosexual difficulties, anxiety and, 214–288

Homosexuality, anxiety and, 169–193

Identification, 54, 118, 135, 142, 213

Intelligence, as criterion for short-term anxiety-provoking psychotherapy, 78, 212

Interaction, *see* Therapist-patient relationship

Interview, *see* Diagnosis; Patients, history of

Knight, R., 115

Konorski, I., 64

Limbic system, 22

Malan, D., 126, 137

Manipulation, acceptable, 24; environmental, 45; excessive pathological, 24

Masochism, 99

Massachusetts General Hospital, Psychiatry Clinic, 11, 76, 138; psychiatry staff, 14, 21

McGuire, M., 95

Medicine, microscopic pathological basis for, 1, 3; relationship with psychiatry, 2–3

Mental health, 24, 31; agency, 32, 33, 34, 35, 37, 41; fellows, 77; professionals, 5

Motivation, 29, 61, 101, 118, 135, 193, 212; as criterion for short-term anxiety-provoking psychotherapy, 84–92 passim; associated with creative process, 90; and curiosity, 86–120 passim, 251

Neurochemistry, 2

Neuropharmacology, 2

Neurophysiology, 2

Nosologies, 2, 22

Obsession, 130

Orthomolecular psychiatry, 22

Index

Paranoia (paranoid), attack, 55; case histories, 51–54; delusions, 55; patients, 36, 50, 55, 56; symptoms, 54; systems, 50

Passivity, enforced, 37; excessive, 99, 115

Patient(s), ability to meet demands, 28; alexithymic, 81; body image, 236, 284; categories, 44, 128; clinging to symptoms, 64; control, 127, 128, 138, 140; expectations of, 95, 97, 100, 122; experimental, 127, 128, 138, 140; history of, 14, 46, 59, 60, 75, 79, 80, 94, 98, 100–102, 224; medication, 56; as a mimic, 134; new, 92; psychotic, 25; schizophrenic, 81; as a victim, 55. *See also* Psychotherapy, brief anxiety-suppressive, selection of patients; Psychotherapy, short-term anxiety-provoking, selection of patients; Therapist-patient relationship

Pauling, L., 22

Phobia, 14, 15, 21, 40, 84, 167, 213; examination, 194–213

Projection, 61, 84, 167; primary, 54, 55; secondary, 54, 55; substitution of, 21

Psychiatrists, 1, 2, 4, 5, 34, 67, 77, 83, 88, 94, 167

Psychiatry, 1–5 passim; clinical, 147, 148, 171, 172, 194, 196, 213, 224; and medicine, 2–4; microscopic, lack of, 1; orthomolecular, 22; scientific trend in, 2. *See also* Resident medical students

Psychodynamic(s), 1, 15 27, 28, 103, 111, 141, 167; case reports, 23–24; continuum, 2, 6, 21–22, 24–25, 27, 29, 43; formulation, 75, 76, 81, 92, 94, 100, 137

Psychological testing, 78

Psychotic breakdown, 34, 57

Psychosomatic medicine, 2, 50

Psychotherapy, conceptual frame of reference for, 6, 44; contradictions of, 82; choice of type needed, 44–45; goal of, 21; intrapsychic changes, 129–135; interpersonal changes, 129–135, 136–143

Psychotherapy, brief anxiety-suppressive, 45–54

Psychotherapy, long-term anxiety-suppressive, 45, 49, 50, 56; case material, 51–56

Psychotherapy, short-term anxiety-provoking, 6, 45, 70–71, 75–92; controlled study of, 127–143; selection of patients, 78–84, 94, 95; evaluation of results, 6, 124–143; evidence of change in, 119–120; examples of technique of, 96–97, 101, 103–104, 105, 109–111, 114, 115, 116, 122; height of treatment in, 99, 109–143, 248; at Massachusetts General Hospital, 76–78; motivation for, 85–92; patient evaualtion, 101–105; problem-solving in, 78, 99, 132–143; psychodynamics of, 75, 93, 123; treatment phases, 105–119. *See also* Therapist-patient relationship

Relationships, 15, 44, 54, 55, 59, 60, 71, 79, 90, 99, 100, 102, 117; meaningful, as criterion for short-term anxiety-provoking psychotherapy, 78, 79, 129, 135. *See also* Therapist-patient relationship

Resident medical students, 3, 77, 93, 102, 116, 117, 121

Sartre, J.-P., 91

Schizophrenia, 22, 81

Schulberg, H. C., 43

Semrad, E. V., 116

Sheldon, A., 43

Silverman, S., 88

Social sciences (scientists), 2, 77

Social workers, 35, 67, 77, 83

Strupp, H., 120

Suicide, 27, 34, 42, 50, 90

Therapist-patient relationship, 93–123; confrontation, 97–99, 112, 113, 143, 242; countertransference, 116–117; encounter, 99–100, psychodynamics, 98–103; 212; transference, 107–109, 152, 158, 212, 236, 239, 248, 257, 259

Thymognosis, 132

Twins, identical, 22